American Dietetic Association Guide to Better Digestion

D1115379

Published by John Wiley & Sons, Inc., Hoboken, New Jersey
Published simultaneously in Canada

Illustrations on pp. 9 and 202 copyright © 2003 by Navta Associates, Inc. All rights reserved

Design and production by Navta Associates, Inc.

Limit of Liability/Disclaimer of Warranty: While the publisher and the author have used their best efforts in preparing this book, they make no representations or warranties with respect to the accuracy or completeness of the contents of this book and specifically disclaim any implied warranties of merchantability or fitness for a particular purpose. No warranty may be created or extended by sales representatives or written sales materials. The advice and strategies contained herein may not be suitable for your situation. You should consult with a professional where appropriate. Neither the publisher nor author shall be liable for any loss of profit or any other commercial damages, including but not limited to special, incidental, consequential, or other damages.

For general information about our other products and services, please contact our Customer Care Department within the United States at (800) 762-2974, outside the United States at (317) 572-3993 or fax (317) 572-4002.

Wiley also publishes its books in a variety of electronic formats. Some content that appears in print may not be available in electronic books. For more information about Wiley products, visit our web site at www.wiley.com.

Library of Congress Cataloging-in-Publication Data:

Bonci, Leslie.
   American Dietetic Association guide to better digestion / Leslie Bonci.
      p. ; cm.
   Includes bibliographical references and index.
      ISBN 0-471-44223-2 (pbk. : alk. paper)
   1. Indigestion—Popular works. 2. Digestion—Popular works.
      [DNLM: 1. Digestive System Diseases—prevention & control—Popular Works.
   2. Digestion—physiology—Popular Works. WI 140 B699a 2003]
   I. Title: Guide to better digestion. II. Title.
   RC827 .B66 2003
   616 . 3—dc21

                                                                2002014016

Printed in the United States of America

10 9 8 7 6 5 4 3 2 1

Contents

Acknowledgments

I t takes a country to write a book, or at least for me it did. My heartfelt thanks to the following individuals for being part of this process.

To Diana Falhauber, my editor at the American Dietetic Association, who gave me the push when I needed it and helped me to cross the finish line.

To Elizabeth Zack, my editor at John Wiley & Sons, whose organizational expertise and insightful comments made this book so reader-friendly.

To the gastroenterologists, especially Dr. Robert Fusco, Dr. Paul Lebovitz, Dr. Arnold Wald, Dr. Steve Lasky, and Dr. Miguel Reguiero for their clinical expertise and willingness to recognize the importance of referring patients to a registered dietitian.

To the countless patients and family members who have shared their stories, exposing very personal accounts of their digestive functions.

To Risa Moldovan, Linda Schorr, and members of the Intestinal Disease Foundation for allowing me to be a board member and peaking my interest in the area of digestive disorders.

To Joy Jenko and members of the Crohn's and Colitis Foundation of America for providing opportunities for me to speak to patients and family members about the very important role of nutrition for good gut health.

To my colleagues, Felicia Busch, M.P.H., R.D., F.A.D.A.; Keith Ayoob, Ed.D., R.D., F.A.D.A.; Althea Zanecosky, M.S., R.D.; and Christine Rosenbloom, Ph.D., R.D. for encouraging me to do this.

With the utmost gratitude to Dr. Freddie Fu, chairman of the Department of Orthopedic Surgery at the University of Pittsburgh Medical Center, for his support and enthusiasm for allowing me writing time.

And most of all, to my family: to my parents for being wonderful role models, and for their insight; to my brother Louis, for his terrific wit and computer proficiency; to my husband Fred, for enduring my mood swings and lending his artistic flair; and to my sons Gregory and Cary, for being good guys and letting mom use the computer to write.

Introduction

In this country, we're obsessed with our guts. Look at the many phrases dealing with the digestive tract that are a regular part of our vocabulary:

- The way to a man's heart is through his stomach.
- That person really has guts.
- I'm following my gut instinct.
- Did you ever feel like you had butterflies in your stomach?

Words such as farting, belching, and gas may be funny to kids, but they're taken very seriously by those who suffer with these symptoms on a regular basis.

When things are working well, the body is remarkably efficient at self-care, and you feel great. But when you are having a bad digestive day, you can feel absolutely miserable.

For example, Diane, a successful therapist in her early thirties, has suffered from constipation since childhood. She sought my help to try to change her bowel habits and lose a little weight. She noted that it was unusual for her to move her bowels more than twice a month. Laughing, but in all seriousness, she said she had clogged her fair share of toilets over the years.

Diane was not a breakfast eater, worked very long hours (with only a quick break to shove lunch in her mouth), and usually had a large dinner at nine or ten at night, and then went to bed. I recommended that she start with a breakfast and build in some snack time during the day. She also agreed to take time for lunch—sitting down and actually eating a meal—and to cut down on the size of her evening meal. After a month of working to change her eating habits, Diane returned for a follow-up grinning from ear to ear. She had been moving her bowels daily, was feeling great, and had even lost a few pounds. In fact, she told me that every time she moves her bowels, she thinks of me!

Whether you suffer from the occasional bout of diarrhea, constipation, heartburn, or abdominal cramps, or have more frequent episodes of abdominal pain and discomfort, you are not alone. Yet, many individuals suffer silently, too embarrassed to discuss their symptoms with a health professional, choosing instead to self-treat. But even though many gastrointestinal disorders are simply more discomforting than life-threatening, you should never self-diagnose, nor should you ignore the symptoms. It's important to be as knowledgeable about your condition as possible. Contact your health care professional, who may refer you to a gastroenterologist, a specialist who can do the appropriate diagnostic tests, so that you can properly manage your symptoms.

In some cases, medications will be prescribed for digestive disorders to help with symptom relief or to prevent other complications. However, it is important to realize that taking care of your gastrointestinal tract is not just about taking a pill. Magazine and television ads may try to sell us on pills or liquids as cure-alls for diarrhea, heartburn, gas, and constipation, but what you eat, your lifestyle habits, and your response to stress are just as important as the medication you may start taking.

American Dietetic Association Guide to Better Digestion is a user-friendly publication focused on dietary modifications, lifestyle habits, and eating survival tips for handling all kinds of gastrointestinal problems. The book is backed by the American Dietetic Association, a professional organization of more than 70,000 registered dietitians and nutrition experts who are important members of the health care team. Understanding the causes and triggers of gastrointestinal disorders can enable you to map out a plan that will help you manage and reduce your uncomfortable symptoms. But even if you are under a physician's care, too often the nutritional advice he or she may offer to help combat your problems is very vague, ranging from "if a certain food bothers you, avoid it" to "eat everything, since food can't help or hurt," to no advice whatsoever. But embarking on the process of making changes in your eating habits and food choices must happen gradually, with a focus on one change at a time. This is not something that can be addressed effectively in one brief office visit. You will find nutritional solutions and practical recommendations on how to implement changes for each disorder in the pages that follow.

This book encourages you to be proactive. After you've read it, you will know what questions to ask your health care professionals and what appropriate referrals to request. You will be informed about your condition, so that you can make a number of changes in your eating habits, food choices, and reaction to stress to diminish the symptoms of your condition. The book also addresses the concerns of caregivers and parents who have questions about how best to take care of loved ones with digestive disorders.

YOUR NUTRITIONAL WELL-BEING

Being well nourished is every individual's right, and even those with gastrointestinal disorders deserve to nourish their bodies optimally. After all, one of the basic requirements of eating is that it be enjoyable. The aroma of a perfectly baked turkey, the visual appeal of a freshly cut watermelon, and the creamy taste of ice cream contribute to the sensory enjoyment of food. Too often, when you have a gastrointestinal disorder, eating is an unpleasant, uncomfortable experience in which you merely "eat to live" instead of relishing your food. This should not be the case. Also, since one of the major functions of food is to nourish the body properly, it is important to find the correct balance regarding food choices and quantities, so that you can make a meal pleasurable and healthful, not painful.

To make an investment in intestinal well-being, one should consider food choices, portions, and meal timing. Food is one of the few things in life that we can control, and it is important to use food in a positive and intestinally friendly way. Experimenting with food choices as well as eating habits can help achieve a more balanced eating pattern, a healthier lifestyle, and, very often, symptom relief.

Other important factors that go a long way toward reducing gastrointestinal upsets include lifestyle variables, such as stress, smoking, and alcohol use. Fitness also plays a very important role in digestive health. These strategies will also be detailed in this book. So whether you have gas or constipation, irritable bowel syndrome or heartburn *American Dietetic Association's Guide to Better Digestion* will define, discuss, and depict nutritional solutions for your digestive disorder.

Having practiced dietetics for twenty years, I have worked with and lectured to hundreds of patients with digestive disorders. I personally have seen and heard that changing food choices and eating behaviors can result in symptom relief; decrease frequency of bowel movements, cramping, nausea, or vomiting; or establishing a regular bowel regime. This can have a profound effect on one's quality of life. It can help enable an individual who was too embarrassed to leave the house for fear of having an "accident" to get out and enjoy life.

Helping people reclaim their lives and enjoy themselves is very gratifying. My goal in writing this book is to enable you to take control, eat well, live well, and feel good.

PART ONE

Understanding Your Digestive System

CHAPTER 1

How Your Gut Works

It is important to have a basic understanding of digestion in order to develop gut-friendly food choices and eating behaviors. Many people think that the process of digestion doesn't begin until food gets into the stomach. It may surprise you to know that digestion begins as soon as the food enters your mouth, and actually even before you start to eat.

Researchers have shown that the taste, texture, smell, and appearance of food may affect the body's ability to absorb nutrients. At the beginning of a meal, even before you start to eat, the brain sends signals to the digestive tract. In the mouth, this results in the secretion of saliva. In the stomach, gastric juices are secreted. In the small intestine, digestive enzymes are released as is the flow of pancreatic juices. If you don't like the way a food looks, smells, or tastes, the body may secrete fewer digestive juices, and the body's ability to move food through the digestive tract may be slower than it would normally be.

To help your body get the maximum benefit from the foods you eat, practice these good eating habits:

- While eating, try to focus on the food, not the TV, computer, or newspaper.

- Take small bites.
- Chew well—don't bite off more than you can chew!
- Eat slowly.
- If you can, sit when you eat, and relax.
- Offer appropriately sized portions to children with digestive disorders.
- If you wear dentures, make sure they fit well, so you can chew foods thoroughly.

Bottom Line

If you want to digest foods well, they should look good, smell good, and taste good. In addition to food choices, good eating habits can add to the enjoyment of a meal.

IN THE MOUTH

What happens to that turkey sandwich you have for lunch? The digestion that occurs in the mouth is both mechanical and chemical. Your teeth and tongue are involved in mechanical digestion, helping you to grind and mix the food to make it easier to swallow. Saliva secreted from salivary glands provides the chemical digestion, which helps to break down foods in the mouth. Three types of saliva are produced in response to different types of foods:

- Salty and bitter foods trigger the production of *salivary amylase,* an enzyme that breaks down starchy foods into sugar. Ever wonder why a piece of bread gets sweeter the longer you chew it? Amylase is the reason.
- Sour foods and fatty foods stimulate production of a type of saliva that makes it easier to swallow larger foods, such as meat.
- Sweets, fruits and vegetables stimulate the production of a type of saliva that dilutes sugar.

The following illustration shows the different parts of the body that are involved in the digestive process. We'll continue to explain how food moves through your system in the pages that follow.

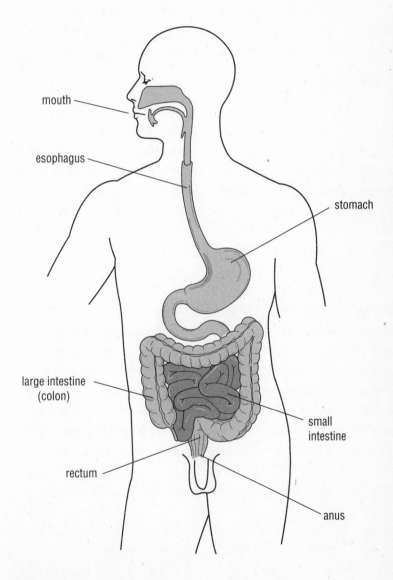

Figure 1.1 – The digestive system

IN THE ESOPHAGUS

After you chew, then swallow, your food, the next stop is the esophagus. This is a ten-inch tube that connects the throat to the stomach and basically acts as a chute to move food from the mouth to the stomach. Muscles in the esophagus move according to a process known as *peristalsis*, contracting and relaxing to push food through.

At the end of the esophagus is the lower esophageal sphincter. This valve is usually closed, but when food comes into contact with it, the valve opens to let the food into the stomach. People who have problems with heartburn or reflux need to pay attention to eating habits and food choices to prevent this sphincter from opening when it shouldn't. If this happens, acid from the stomach can flow up into the esophagus, causing the sensation of heartburn. (For more information on heartburn, refer to chapter 5.)

IN THE STOMACH

If you have ever said, "My eyes are larger than my stomach!" you haven't been able to finish your food because you have felt full. Although the stomach can hold quite a lot (up to one gallon of food and liquid combined when fully stretched), there is an upper limit of comfort. The stomach basically acts like a mixer, breaking food into smaller pieces and adding digestive juices to allow for easier absorption. Muscles of the stomach contract to blend food, while the gastric juices and enzymes that are produced in the stomach further break down food. This mixture is then pushed through the end of the stomach to the pyloric valve, which is located at the duodenum, or top of the small intestine. This valve allows only one teaspoon of food at a time to enter the duodenum. Full emptying of the stomach can take anywhere from two hours for a regular-size meal to four hours for a high-fat meal, such as fried chicken or a pepperoni pizza.

IN THE SMALL INTESTINE

The small intestine is where most of the digestion of food occurs. Whole foods are broken down into nutrients: protein, carbohydrate, and fat. The digestive juices secreted from the small intestine are assisted by:

- Digestive enzymes secreted from the pancreas, which break the food down into protein, carbohydrate, and fat.
- Bile, a solution produced by the liver that helps digest fat.
- A more concentrated form of bile, which is stored in the gallbladder and released into the small intestine when you eat fat-containing foods.

The carbohydrate, protein, and fat are then further broken down to metabolites, byproducts of digestion, which can be absorbed through the intestine into the blood stream to the liver cells. There, they can be used for various body functions. Water, vitamins, and minerals from food are also absorbed here. In fact, the majority of nutrient absorption takes place in the upper portion of the small intestine.

To illustrate this process, the turkey sandwich with mayonnaise that you had for lunch might become the following:

Food	Nutrient		Metabolites
Bread	carbohydrate	→	saccharides → glucose (energy)
Turkey	protein	→	amino acids
Mayonnaise	fat	→	triglycerides → fatty acids + glycerol

In the small intestine, digestion occurs slowly, with a little bit of food at a time. Food moves through to the second part of the small intestine, the jejunum, and through to the ileum, which absorbs vitamin B_{12} and also bile acids from the liver and gallbladder. This movement and digestion of food in the small intestine can last from thirty minutes to three hours.

IN THE LARGE INTESTINE

The large intestine, or colon, is the waste removal system for the body. The remaining components of digestion—water, fiber, sodium, and potassium—that have not been used by the body enter the colon through the ileocecal valve. Water is removed through absorption. The leftover components, or stool (fiber, bacteria, and dead cells from the lining of the digestive tract), moves through the colon by muscular contractions to the anus, or rectum, where it will be eliminated through the anal sphincter. This process can take from twelve to twenty-four hours.

The process of digestion involves the entire digestive tract from mouth to anus. What you eat, and how much, can shorten or lengthen the time it takes for food to pass through your body. Now we will learn what happens when things go wrong with various parts of the digestive process, and more important, what you can do to have optimal digestion.

CHAPTER 2

Survival Skills for Self-Managing Your Digestive Condition

When you have a digestive disorder, whether it's constipation, irritable bowel syndrome (IBS), gas, or diarrhea, often just getting through the day can sap all your energy and enthusiasm. Part of learning how to self-manage any intestinal disorder is developing good "gut survival skills," which concentrate on four areas: appropriate food choices, eating behaviors, lifestyle activities, and stress management. We'll concentrate on these in a moment.

One of the difficulties of intestinal illnesses is that you can be doing all the right things, and still have days when you don't feel good. Be assured that you haven't done anything wrong. There will be some rough roads along the way, so just take advantage of the days you feel well. On the days you don't—relax, regroup, and give yourself a chance to rest.

To be your most successful, however, you need to make attending to your digestive health a priority. We all have obligations to work, family, and friends; often our own needs are at the bottom of the priority list. But no one else can make the changes for you, and only you are going to be able to tell what works and what doesn't. I am going to ask you to make a commitment—not to me, family, or friends—but to *yourself.* If you want to feel good, you need to make the time to find out what works, and what doesn't, in terms of your gut. This isn't being selfish, but self-caring.

APPROPRIATE FOOD AND BEVERAGE CHOICES

Listen to your own body; everyone responds differently to food items. So don't assume that because your friend who also has ulcerative colitis (see chapter 7) can't tolerate dairy products that you can't either. Also, when you get yourself into the mindset that there are "good" versus "bad" foods, it can jeopardize your nutritional well-being. Eliminating too many foods from a diet can mean that you are not getting the proper nourishment. Also, you may classify some foods, such as fruits and vegetables, as "good," but while these *are* very good for health, they also may be hard to digest. If the only vegetables you can eat are those that are well cooked, don't worry too much about it; you still get nutritional benefits, even if some of the nutrients are lost through the cooking process. In addition, you may think you are being "bad" when you eat foods you consider "bad," or think that eating those foods will somehow worsen your digestive disorder. Don't beat yourself up this way. Food is essential for survival, and eating should be a pleasant experience for you, not one that causes you stress.

In fact, one of the goals of eating is to achieve as balanced and varied a diet as you can. This is not only good for your gut, but benefits the rest of your body as well. No one food provides all the nutrients the body needs. Different kinds of foods provide different nutrients to the body. The Food Guide Pyramid details the types and amounts of foods to include daily for a healthy, balanced diet. If you have a digestive disorder, you will want to customize the pyramid to include foods and portions that you can best tolerate.

For the body to be well nourished, you must include the three energy sources in your diet every day: carbohydrate, protein, and fat.

Carbohydrates are found in foods such as bread, cereal, rice, pasta,

Food Guide Pyramid
A Guide to Daily Food Choices

KEY

◻ Fat (naturally occurring and added)
◩ Sugars (added)

These symbols show fat and added sugars in foods.
They come mostly from the fats, oils, and sweets group.
But foods in other groups—such as cheese or ice cream
from the milk group or french fries from the vegetable
group—can also provide fat and added sugars.

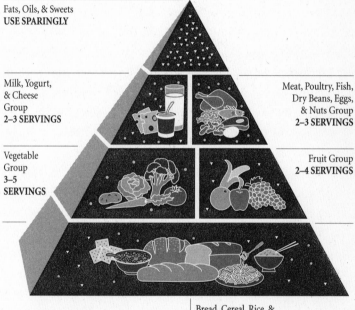

Fats, Oils, & Sweets
USE SPARINGLY

Milk, Yogurt,
& Cheese
Group
2–3 SERVINGS

Meat, Poultry, Fish,
Dry Beans, Eggs,
& Nuts Group
2–3 SERVINGS

Vegetable
Group
**3–5
SERVINGS**

Fruit Group
2–4 SERVINGS

Bread, Cereal, Rice, &
Pasta Group
6–11 SERVINGS

Source: USDA and DHHS

crackers, fruits, vegetables, and sweets. These foods provide energy
to the body, and are foods that many of us like to eat. It is a good
idea to try to include some type of carbohydrate-containing food at
every meal and snack.

Protein is found in meat, poultry, fish, eggs, dairy products, nuts,
seeds, soy foods, and dried beans. Protein is important for muscle
growth and repair, and to support a healthy immune system. Try to
include some protein at every meal and snack.

Fat, found in foods such as oil, nuts, spreads, and salad dressings, is a source of energy for the body. Fat also gives flavor to food, and certain types of fats found in fish, nuts, and oils such as olive, canola, peanut, and safflower oil can be very good for heart health. A small amount of fat goes a long way to add to the enjoyment of a meal, and you should make sure it is part of yours.

So what should comprise an ideal plate of food? Picture your plate as a peace sign. Protein should take up one-third of the plate, and carbohydrate should be the remainder of the plate, with half coming from a starchy food (bread, cereal, rice, and pasta) and the other half from a fruit or vegetable. What about fat, then? Fat is typically consumed in smaller quantities than protein and carbohydrate, and may be included as a component of a protein food, such as cheese or nuts, or as an addition to a food, such as olive oil used to sauté vegetables, or margarine added to a baked potato.

Not only what you eat, but the *form* of food you eat may have an effect on your gut. I have had patients tell me that they feel they are cheating if they eat canned fruits and vegetables or white bread instead of whole wheat. You have to listen to your body. Canned fruits or vegetables still provide your body with nutritional benefits, and may be easier to digest than fresh fruits. Whole grain food is very nutritious, but if it causes pain, there is no point in suffering. White bread, white rice, or a corn or rice cereal will still provide the body with valuable carbohydrates.

Variety is also an important component of your diet. To get the proper nutrition, you will want to consider adding new foods to your diet even if you have a digestive disorder. However, when I recommend new foods for patients to try, I always remind them that the first time they try a new food it may not work. If that happens, don't say, "I'll never eat that food again," but try it again *in a few days*. When you add a new food, just add one new food at a time, in a very small amount, and make that the only new thing you try that day. You can gradually increase the amount if your system begins to tolerate it. I have also had people with digestive diseases say that they try to eat the recommended number of servings of fruits and vegetables a day and feel that they have failed when they find they can't tolerate that volume of produce. For many fruits and vegetables, the recommended serving is half a cup. However, someone with a digestive disease may only be able to handle a serving size of one tablespoon! Remember, this is not a race. You don't have to compare yourself to anyone else. *It is always better to start small and gradually add one more bite at a time.*

In addition to appropriate food choices, it is also important to get enough fluids. If you don't drink enough, you may feel more tired and more uncomfortable. As with food, it is important to find what works best for you in terms of fluid choices and amounts. Very often, my well-intentioned patients try to boost their fluid intake drastically, only to find that they are spending more time in the bathroom than they did before.

In order to achieve the goal of being well hydrated and feeling comfortable, you need to figure out what your fluid requirements are and establish a drinking schedule to follow. Fluid needs are based on body weight and activity level. In general, the amount of fluid needed on a daily basis is one of the following:

Body weight (pounds) × 0.5 = Number of ounces of fluid if you don't exercise regularly

Body weight (pounds) × 0.67 = Number of ounces of fluid if you do exercise regularly

As a first step, figure out what your needs are according to your weight and activity level. Then, record your fluid intake for a typical day. The goal is to establish a routine that will gradually boost your fluid intake by no more than one cup at a time. A good strategy is to add one cup of fluid a day for one week, and then add another cup of fluid for the second week, until you meet your goal.

Keep in mind that fluids include everything you drink, such as water, juice, milk, decaffeinated products, and sports drinks.

Certain fluids, such as those containing caffeine, and herbs such as guarana, maté, and kola nut, may stress your digestive tract. Some people find that carbonated beverages can be irritating, and they may make you feel full before your fluid requirements are met. Alcohol can irritate the digestive tract of certain people, and may also cause fluid loss. If your beverage of choice is fruit juice, you may need to experiment to find the kinds that feel most comfortable to your gut.

Don't forget that certain foods also contribute to your fluid intake. Fruits and vegetables are 90 to 95 percent water. Liquid foods, such as soup, gelatin, and frozen products such as fruit ices, and popsicles, can also be fluid sources, and they provide some variety. Here is how one patient of mine successfully boosted his fluid intake.

Jim, who suffered from constipation, was told to increase his fluid intake. In the past, he had tried adding several glasses of water to his daily meals, but spent so much time in the bathroom that he wasn't able to keep up with this plan. Jim weighed 175 pounds and exercised three to four times a week. His fluid needs were 175×0.67, or approximately 117 ounces of fluid per day.

After keeping track of his beverage intake, Jim figured out that he was consuming about 60 ounces of fluid a day. He decided to make gradual changes in his drinking schedule as follows:

Week 1: 68 ounces of fluid a day

Week 2: 76 ounces of fluid a day

Week 3: 84 ounces of fluid a day

Week 4: 90 ounces of fluid a day

Week 5: 98 ounces of fluid a day

Week 6: 106 ounces of fluid a day

Week 7: 114 ounces of fluid a day

By week 4, Jim noticed an improvement in his bowel habits. By week 8, he was able to move his bowels every day, and he even noticed improved energy levels during the day as a result of drinking enough.

Making the Right Food Choices in Unusual Situations

Being in control of your food choices and eating situations can be a very positive feeling. It is usually easy to control eating in your own home, but what do you do when you go out? Here are some guidelines to help when you are away from home.

- Ask questions about the food choices and make requests.
- Bring snacks when traveling by car or plane.
- If you are traveling by air, call ahead to learn what types of special meals are served.
- If you are dining out in a new restaurant, call ahead to see what the chef can do to make your meal gut-friendly.
- Ask what ingredients are in a particular food item or sauce.
- Ask if an item can be prepared without added fats.
- Ask if the vegetables can be cooked well.
- Travel with a food survival kit that includes crackers, packets of hot cereal (you can always get hot water), tea bags, small cans of fruit nectar, small cans of fruit or applesauce, and dry soup mix.
- Call ahead to the hotel to ask about the availability of an in-room refrigerator, microwave, or hot plate.
- For a long stay, find a local store to stock up on some favorite foods.
- When traveling to a non-English-speaking country, contact the language department of your local university to see if someone can translate a list of your food preferences and intolerances, or search the Internet for this type of information.

Bottom Line _____

- Include a mix of nutrients and food groups at each meal.
- Start with a small amount of a new food.
- Only add one new food at a time.
- Try a new food more than once.
- Include a beverage, or liquid food, with every meal and snack.

If you notice any changes as a result of making new food and beverage choices, it is important to note any changes in gastrointestinal symptoms, such as changes in bowel habits and abdominal pain. Keep track of these changes in your food diary (see chapter 3), noting whether the symptoms are improving, staying the same, or getting worse. You may also notice some benefits seemingly unrelated to gut health, including higher energy levels, improved sleep patterns, or a better mood. Document these in your food diary as well.

Abigail, a delightful eight-year-old with Crohn's disease, which is an inflammatory condition of the digestive tract (see chapter 7), has a social schedule that would tire an adult. In addition to playing sports year round, she is always being invited to parties, sleepovers and all-day outings with friends and family. There are many foods that she does not tolerate well, but that doesn't stop her from having a great time.

On the following page are some suggestions to help your child be prepared for any social activity.

EATING BEHAVIORS

To be as gut-friendly as possible, you should pay attention not only to making the appropriate food choices, but to the way you eat. With today's busy lives, it is a rarity to be able to sit down to a nice relaxing meal. So it is important to discover what your own eating

Making Sure Your Child Has the Right Foods in Unusual Situations

- Encourage your child to bring along a stash of friendly tummy goodies, and enough to share as well.
- If your child is going to a party, you may want to call the parents ahead of time and explain your child's situation.
- Keep acceptable foods in the car, and make sure you put some in your child's backpack or sports bag.

habits are like. Do you eat quickly or slowly? Do you chew your food well, or take big bites? Do you sip or gulp beverages? If you rush through meals, chances are you may feel more uncomfortable after eating.

Here are some wise new behavior strategies to follow if you want to reduce the risk of upsetting your gut:

- First and foremost, make eating purposeful. When you eat *just eat.* If you are at your computer, in your car, watching television, or talking on the phone, your attention is not on the food, because you are distracted. You may be more likely to eat more quickly when you are distracted. In addition, if you are stuck in traffic, watching something upsetting on television, or in the process of accidentally deleting a document on your computer while you eat, your digestive tract may pay the price.
- Take small bites and chew thoroughly so you can really taste your food.
- Sip beverages instead of gulping.
- Take the time to eat.
- Sit down to eat a meal or snack instead of eating at the kitchen sink or behind the wheel of your car.
- Eat smaller amounts of food at a time, spacing meals and snacks at regular intervals throughout the day. This is much

more comfortable for the gut, and provides an added benefit of more energy throughout the day.

It is important to work on making your eating environment and food choices gut-friendly, and find out what works best for you and your family.

Bottom Line

- Eating habits are just as important as food choices.
- Space food throughout the day.
- Eating should be a priority, not an afterthought.
- Make mealtime a relaxing experience.

LIFESTYLE STRATEGIES

It is very important to address other aspects of a healthy lifestyle when trying to solve digestive problems. Physical activity can help with symptom management, primarily because it can serve as a distraction. Going out for a walk, swimming, or riding a bicycle makes you focus on the exercise, not your colon. Any type of exercise that you find enjoyable will work well.

Too often, people with digestive disorders adopt a more sedentary lifestyle because they are afraid that exercise will worsen symptoms, or that they may not be able to get to a bathroom in time. Yet physical activity is good for the heart, lungs, and muscles, not just for the gut.

Ease into any physical activity gradually. If you haven't exercised in a while, start small, five to ten minutes, and build from there. You also may want to consider doing some strength training with weights. For this more controlled exercise you can stand in one place, so it may be less stressful to your gut. Stretching and flexibility exercises are also very calming to the body and do not stress your digestive tract. If you have never tried yoga, Pilates, or T'ai C'hi, you may find these exercises to be quite fun and soothing to your gastrointestinal tract as well.

It is also important to time your exercise so that you don't cause digestive distress. Give yourself a chance to relax and digest your food before you exercise. Vigorous movement too close to mealtimes can cause food to move through your intestines more quickly, resulting in more rapid bowel movements.

For example, Carol was always active, playing sports in college and enjoying a lifetime of biking, hiking, and swimming with her husband John. After retiring from a teaching career, she and John (also retired) intended to enjoy life. Then Carol was diagnosed with ulcerative colitis, which required surgery. After surgery left her with chronic diarrhea, she worried that she would not be able to exercise regularly, for fear of not being able to get to a bathroom in time. John, her husband, came up with a solution. He bought Carol a cell phone, so that when she goes out for walk or bike ride, she can contact him quickly if she is not near a restroom. Carol hasn't slowed down yet!

In fact, she never turns down an opportunity to exercise. She just makes sure her cell phone is with her, and out she goes, knowing that if she feels the urge to go and needs to get to a bathroom quickly, John will come to the rescue.

Bottom Line

- Add exercise gradually.
- Do activities you like.
- Wait a while after eating before you exercise.
- Do some strength training.
- Focus on exercise for your heart, such as walking, bicycling, or swimming, and for your muscles.
- Include stretching exercises, too, such as T'ai C'hi, yoga, or Pilates.

STRESS MANAGEMENT STRATEGIES

When it comes to stress management, the issue is not the stress itself, but how we respond to it. If you notice that you experience pain in your stomach or gut when you are upset, angry, or happy, you may benefit from incorporating stress reduction techniques into your daily routine.

I vividly remember walking home after school as a child, coming into the house, and seeing my mother on the floor with her legs resting on the wall. This was always a sign that she didn't want to be bothered. Many years later, I asked her why she would do that. She said that when she was "on the wall" she couldn't do anything else, and it was her way to unwind. She still does it today!

There are many other ways to unwind and de-stress, however. Some people employ the technique of visualization: they close their eyes, imagine a favorite place, and immediately relax. Some people put on soothing music or slip into an inviting bubble bath. Others simply sit for a few minutes, enjoying a little peace and quiet, before they leave the office for the day to encounter traffic or deal with issues at home. For some, the smell of lavender, eucalyptus, or peppermint can be very soothing.

What works for you? It doesn't matter if it is any or all of these situations, just make sure you work in some "time-out" time for you. This may seem like an indulgence, and you may feel there is too much to do, but let's face it—the emails, dishes, chores, homework, and bills will still be there, and you will be in a much better frame of mind to attend to them after you have had a little quiet time for yourself.

If you are not currently putting some quiet time into your day, you may need a daily reminder so that it can become a habit. Relaxation time should be part of the to-do list just as work, social, and family obligations are. So write a note to yourself in your appointment book or PalmPilot, or put a note beside the phone or on your refrigerator. A little downtime can do wonders for your gut.

It also helps if after meals you sit, relax, and give yourself a chance to enjoy what you have eaten. If you are experiencing some discomfort after eating, try resting a hot water bottle, wrapped in a towel, on your abdominal area. Try not to sit down to a meal when you are pressed for time; you won't enjoy your food, and may have more symptoms. If you need to dash out the door to a meeting, or to take a child to sports practice, put the meal on hold. Just have a small snack and wait until you have time to actually sit uninterrupted to eat a full meal.

Children with inflammatory bowel diseases should also try to get into the habit of sitting after meals, or having a little quiet time to allow foods to digest. This takes practice, and can be very hard for the child who is used to rushing around. So sit with your children after meals, perhaps to read a story or just talk.

Establish a support network. Suffering silently is never the solution, whereas seeking support of a few family members and close friends, or through a group situation, can help you through the tough times, as well as provide a psychological and emotional lift. Educate and inform colleagues and teachers about your situation, or your child's digestive disorder. For example, children with inflammatory bowel diseases may find it necessary to leave the classroom in the middle of a class to go to the bathroom. It is better to explain your child's situation to the teacher at the beginning of the school year, to prevent embarrassment when the need for a quick bathroom trip arises.

Ann's son Noah was diagnosed with Crohn's disease. He was a very active six-year-old who never wanted to sit still. After snacks and lunch at school, he would have to go to the bathroom several times. When concerned notes from Noah's teacher started arriving, Ann went in to talk to her. The teacher switched story time to after lunch, and art projects to after snacks. These more relaxed and pleasant activities worked to reduce the number of bathroom trips Noah needed, and there were no more notes from school.

Bottom Line

- Engage in activities that are relaxing to you.
- If your child has a digestive disorder, be a good role model and relax with him or her after eating.
- Schedule some quiet time after meals.
- Delay meals if you are too rushed to be able to enjoy your food.
- Make stress reduction a daily occurrence.
- Don't be afraid to seek support.

Developing good survival skills can be of benefit for *any* digestive disorder. Putting yourself in the equation is the first step toward good gut health. Learning how, what, and when to eat can help you to fuel your body appropriately. Exercising can help you feel refreshed, reinvigorated, and take your mind off your gut. Stress reduction techniques will help you feel relaxed and renewed. Make all of these strategies a part of your daily routine for your intestinal, physical, emotional, and mental well-being.

CHAPTER 3

Getting Started

One of the first steps toward achieving optimal digestion is getting an idea of what your current eating pattern looks like. You can then start working toward a meal plan that will allow you to achieve optimal digestion much of the time. Start by creating a food diary: record what you eat each day in a small notebook, a spread sheet on your computer, or the form you'll find later in this chapter. To get the most out of tracking your eating patterns, try to keep a food diary for at least one week, recording for each day the following information:

Detailed information about the food you eat
- Time that you eat or drink.
- What you eat or drink, with as much detail as possible.
- Brand names of any packaged food consumed.
- Portion size—the amount that you actually ate or drank. (To estimate portion sizes, use your hand as a guide, for example, a palm-size serving of meat, or a fist-size serving of pasta or rice.)
- How the food was prepared—grilled, fried, baked, and so forth.
- What you added to the food, for example, seasonings, condiments, butter, salad dressings, or jelly.

- Supplements, such as vitamins and minerals, herbs, and protein powders.

Activities engaged in while eating
- Talking on the phone
- Standing
- Sitting at the table
- Working at the computer
- Reading
- Driving

Digestive symptoms (Record this information in a different colored pen or pencil, or a different font next to the food or foods you think are causing the problem.)
- Abdominal pain or bloating
- Diarrhea
- Nausea or vomiting

The table opposite is an example of what a sample filled-in food diary can look like. A blank food diary page follows so you can start to fill it out. You'll find more blank food diary pages at the end of the book.

ANALYZING THE INFORMATION

Recording this information can help identify foods that cause unpleasant reactions, and problem eating habits, such as infrequent or large meals, and can help you put together an eating plan that works for you. But remember that just recording one day's worth of information isn't enough. Try to record at least a week's worth of eating. Once your food diary is complete, you'll want to use the information you compiled to develop a list of the following:

- Potential food triggers—foods or beverages that trigger uncomfortable gastrointestinal symptoms

SAMPLE FOOD DIARY

Time	Food	Amount	Activities	Symptoms
7 A.M.	Cheerios	1 cup	Standing at the sink	Felt okay
	2% milk	½ cup		
	Banana	½ of 5-inch		
8 A.M.	Tea, black, plain	10-oz mug	In the car	Rumbling
9 A.M.			At office desk	Gassy
9:15 A.M.			Rushing to bathroom	Diarrhea
10 A.M.	Water	3 gulps	At desk	A little queasy
11 A.M.			Answering phone	Nauseous
12 noon	Turkey sandwich: Turkey breast— deli	4 bites 2 slices	At the computer	Uncomfortable
	White bread— bakery	2 slices		
	Mayonnaise	1 tbsp.		
12:30			Rushing to bathroom	Diarrhea
1 P.M.	Water	8-oz glass	Sitting at desk	A little queasy
2 P.M.	Tea, black, plain	12-oz mug	Relaxing at desk	Better
3 P.M.	Applesauce, sweetened	4-oz carton	Working at desk	Okay
4 P.M.	Ginger ale	½ can	On the phone	Bloated
5 P.M.			Driving home	Gassy
5:30 P.M.			Lying on sofa	Bloated
6 P.M.	Chicken breast, skinless, baked, fat-free dressing	palm-size	At the dining room table	Okay
	White rice, plain	½ cup		
	Green beans, canned, plain	2 tbsp.		
	Lemonade, from powder	8-oz glass		
7 P.M.			Watching TV news	Okay
8 P.M.	Fruit ice	½ cup	Paying bills	A little abdominal pain
9 P.M.	Water	4-oz glass	In bed	Feeling better

YOUR PERSONAL FOOD DIARY

Time	Food	Amount	Activities	Symptoms

- Foods that seem to be safe for you to eat
- Times when you seem to have the most digestive problems, for example, at a certain time of day or after large meals
- Eating habits that contribute to your discomfort

My food and beverage triggers

_____

_____

_____

_____

_____

_____

My safe foods

_____

_____

_____

_____

_____

Troublesome times of the day

_____

_____

_____

_____

_____

Bothersome eating habits

_____

_____

_____

_____

_____

Analyzing the information you collect can help you identify potentially troublesome foods, more difficult times of the day for you, or eating habits that can contribute to your discomfort, such as eating too fast or eating too much at one time. Yet, as helpful as it can be to have a record of what you are doing, be aware that there may be times when a food or beverage that is normally fine for you to consume is suddenly bothersome for no apparent reason. That can happen to anyone. Still, monitoring food intake can help you construct a list of gut-friendly foods that do not cause symptoms and can be labeled as your "safe foods."

It is a good idea to keep your list of safe foods in a place where you can easily find it—perhaps on the refrigerator or taped inside the pantry door. These items should become known as your "food survival list." Keep not only a list of favorite foods, but also foods you turn to when you don't feel well or when you want to reduce the odds of stomach upsets. Start a list of these safe foods now. If possible, keep these items on hand in your glove compartment, purse, briefcase, or office desk. For children with digestive disorders, put a few of their "safe" comfort foods in the knapsack, gym bag, school locker, or desk. For younger children, give the food items to the teacher or child-care personnel.

Food Survival List

Favorite foods

_____

_____

_____

_____

Foods I choose when I don't feel well

_____

_____

_____

_____

MODIFYING EATING PATTERNS

In addition to keeping track of food choices, timing of meals, and activities while eating, it is also a good idea to record your eating patterns with the following information:

- How quickly do you eat? Record the time spent.
- Do you eat only when hungry, or for other reasons? For example, do you grab a snack when someone else is eating, or buy a cookie when you pass a bakery even though you just finished lunch?
- Do you eat until comfortable or full? Rate yourself on a scale of one to five, with one being still hungry after eating a meal, and five being uncomfortably full.

The table on the following page is an example of how to record information about eating patterns:

By recording your eating patterns, you will be able to determine whether more of your eating occurs when you are truly hungry, or for nonhunger reasons. The goal is to eat in response to hunger. To achieve better gastrointestinal comfort, you will want to stop eating when satisfied, but not overly full. Keeping track of your eating patterns will allow you to identify why you eat and how quickly you eat, so that you can start to modify your current eating behaviors. You will also be able to note whether you make a lot of changes in your diet at once, or only change one item at a time. After all, *how* you eat is just as important as *what* you eat.

MOVING TOWARD A MEAL PLAN
THAT WORKS FOR YOU

Identifying problem foods, emphasizing safe foods, and gradually modifying your diet over time can decrease the apprehension you may feel when it comes time to eat, and increase the likelihood for success with regards to gastrointestinal symptom relief and improved

Sample Record of Eating Patterns

Time Eaten	Food	Rate of Eating	Eaten for Hunger or Other Reason	Rating of Fullness (1 to 5; 1—still hungry, 5—very full)
12 noon	Hamburger on bun	5 minutes	H	1
	12-oz Coke	5 minutes	H	1
	Apple	3 minutes	H	2
	Potato chips, 1-oz bag	2 minutes	H	3
12:30 P.M.	Piece of birthday cake	2 minutes	O—co-worker's birthday party	4
12:30 P.M.	2 cookies	3 minutes	O—party	5
2:00 P.M.	Handful of chips	5 minutes	H	3
2:00 P.M.	12-oz Coke	10 minutes	H	5

Your Personal Record of Eating Patterns

Time Eaten	Food	Rate of Eating	Eaten for Hunger or Other Reason	Rating of Fullness (1 to 5; 1—still hungry, 5—very full)

nutritional well-being. But bear in mind that food avoidance, or being overly restrictive about what you can eat, can have negative effects on your physical and emotional well-being. Eating should provide pleasure, not pain, so try to make it a positive experience. Also, when trying to modify your eating patterns, set small, attainable goals with an emphasis on increasing your tolerance to a particular food, or changing the speed at which you eat. This can be easier to accomplish and maintain than an all-or-nothing approach. In the pages that follow, we'll discuss the most common digestive disorders and recommend ways to alter your meal plans and make other lifestyle changes so that you can find symptom relief.

Realize that what ultimately works best for you can be entirely different than the approach that might be best for someone else. And remember: food can, and should, be comforting to the body.

Cautionary Words About Supplement Use

You may have read, seen, or heard about a supplement that could be helpful for your digestive disorder. Although the majority of these products are available over-the-counter, there are some facts about supplements that are worth mentioning:

- Supplements should never be considered a replacement for establishing healthy food choices and eating behaviors.
- Supplements are not "one size fits all." You may find a particular product to be helpful or to be no help at all.
- Do inform your physician and dietitian of any supplement you decide to try, especially if you are on medications.
- The herbal supplements listed in this book are those that have been approved by the German Commission E monograph, a compilation of research studies that test herbs for safety. However, the *efficacy* of a particular herb is not tested. If you are going to try any herb, select

from the ones that are listed in the following chapters. These herbs are referenced in the *PDR for Herbal Medicines, 2000.*

- In the United States, supplement use is not regulated by the Food and Drug Administration (FDA). Therefore, the purity of a product is not guaranteed as it is in Germany. The dosage, quality, and actual ingredients of a product can vary widely from brand to brand.

- Recognize that "natural" and "safe" are not synonymous terms. A product with the word "natural" on the label can still be dangerous, or can worsen symptoms.

- The nonherbal supplements listed in this book are based on the *PDR for Nutritional Supplements, 2001,* a professional reference that provides a research summary for products listed. Some of these supplements have been more extensively tested than others, and again, if you are going to try one, do be aware that the quality of a product is not always guaranteed. If there is a particular supplement that sounds intriguing, your best bet is to use the brand that is cited in the PDR reference.

- Do not exceed the dose recommended on the product label.

- Do not try more than one product simultaneously.

- If you experience any unusual side effects, discontinue the use of these supplements immediately and call your physician!

- Do not give supplements to children. The one exception is a vitamin-mineral supplement, or a specific supplement that your doctor may prescribe.

- Women who are pregnant or nursing should not take supplements except for a prenatal vitamin-mineral supplement, or a specific vitamin or mineral formulation that your doctor feels is necessary.

PART TWO

Moving toward Better Digestion

CHAPTER 4

Food-borne Illnesses and Prevention

D riving home from a bridge tournament, my brother Louis decided to stop at a roadside restaurant for a bite to eat. He ordered a turkey dinner that he said was quite tasty, and, feeling satisfied, he got back in his car to drive home. The next evening, he called to say that he was having diarrhea, and was also vomiting. He asked my husband and father to come to his apartment. When they arrived, Louis was lying on the floor, and seemed confused. They took him to the hospital where tests confirmed that he had Shigella, a food-borne bacteria. After receiving IV fluids, he was sent home to recuperate. Needless to say, Louis has crossed that restaurant off his list!

WHAT IS FOOD-BORNE ILLNESS?

Food-borne illness may affect up to 76 million Americans every year. Although food poisoning is not a digestive disease, the symptoms are gastrointestinal. If you have ever had food poisoning, it is an experience you won't soon forget. As the body uses every measure to get rid of the food toxins, the affected person may make frequent trips to the bathroom, alternating between diarrhea and vomiting. The good news is that the suffering is relatively short, and for the most part, food poisoning can be prevented by practicing proper food handling techniques.

Food poisoning is caused by the harmful bacteria that are found in foods that are outdated, subjected to germs in handling, improperly stored, or not cooked to the right temperature. The following table lists the different types of food-borne pathogens. Most food poisoning is a result of eating protein-containing foods that have been improperly cooked. This is why it is so important to cook foods thoroughly. However, sometimes produce, too, can harbor bacteria that can make you ill, so you should always wash fruits and vegetables well before eating.

Food-borne Illnesses

Food Source	Pathogens
Raw, undercooked meat and poultry	Campylobacter jejuni, E. coli, L. monocytogenes, Salmonella
Unpasteurized milk and dairy products	L. monocytogenes, Salmonella, Shigella, Staphylococcus aureus, C. jejuni
Raw or undercooked eggs	Salmonella
Raw or undercooked shellfish	Vibrio vulnificus, Vibrio parahaemolyticus
Improperly canned products	C. botulinum
Produce	E. coli, L. monoctogenes, Salmonella, Shigella, Yersinia enterocolitica

There are control measures in place in the grocery stores and restaurants to keep food safe, but you need to take similar precautions at home as well. A few minutes spent on thorough handwashing and correct food handling can keep your digestive system free of food-borne bacteria. If you already have digestive disorders, it is doubly important for you to practice food safety, since the majority of symptoms of food poisoning negatively affect the gut. The symptoms include:

- Abdominal cramps
- Nausea
- Vomiting
- Diarrhea
- Fever
- Dehydration

Although symptoms typically resolve on their own, you should contact your doctor if you are experiencing any of the following symptoms:

- Weak or rapid pulse
- Shallow breathing
- Cold, clammy, pale skin
- Shaking or chills
- Chest pain
- Symptoms of severe dehydration, such as dry mouth, decreased urine output, sunken eyes, low blood pressure
- Confusion

PREVENTING FOOD POISONING

To prevent as much as possible incidents of food poisoning, adopt a safe food handling program in your own food preparation. The Fight Bac, and Home Food Safety campaigns are designed to keep you and your food safe. (See appendix F for contact information.) You'll also want to take precautions in the grocery store, while preparing and serving food, and in storing leftovers. First, let's highlight the four key points of the Home Food Safety Campaign.

1. Wash hands thoroughly with soap and water before handling food—for twenty seconds, or two verses of "Happy Birthday." You also need to wash hands before and after handling raw meats.
2. Keep hot foods hot (use a meat thermometer).

3. Keep cold foods cold (store at proper temperatures and in appropriate containers).
4. Keep raw and cooked food separate with two sets of cutting boards and utensils.

You may prefer a plastic cutting board instead of a wooden one. Both are fine, but either should be thrown away if there are gouges in the surface where bacteria can hide. Cutting boards need to be cleaned after every use with hot soapy water. If your cutting board is plastic, put it through the dishwasher as often as possible.

BUYING FOODS

When you are buying foods, always have a food safety strategy in mind:

- In the produce aisle, select fruits and vegetables that are not bruised or moldy.
- See what you buy—choose loose produce, instead of packaged, whenever possible.
- Buy only juices that are pasteurized.
- In the cereal aisle, make sure boxes are tightly sealed, and check the expiration date.
- Buy only cans that are not dented or bulging.
- Buy perishables last—meat, poultry, fish, eggs, milk, cheeses, and frozen foods.
- Be a detective—make sure packages are tightly sealed.
- Look for the Safe Food Handling label that is now displayed on packaged meats, and follow the instructions on this label to properly handle your meats.
- Check expiration dates!
- Put meats in the basket away from other foods, and have the bagger pack meats separately. Put leaky meats in the plastic bags found in the produce aisle to keep them away from the rest of the food in your basket.

- If you will be away from home longer than one hour, keep a cooler in your trunk with ice packs, and put the perishable foods in there.
- If you are buying hot, ready-to-eat foods, and will not be eating them within one hour, reheat them when you get to your final destination.

FOOD SAFETY AT HOME

A little effort to follow these guidelines can pay off in a big way to keep you safe and your gut happy. When you get home:

- Refrigerate perishable foods first!
- Keep eggs in the original carton, and store in the coldest part of the refrigerator (not on the refrigerator door).
- Don't store milk on the door.
- Put meat on the bottom shelf of the refrigerator in the back, or in the freezer, in freezer wrap, with a date on the wrapping.
- Make sure your refrigerator is at the proper temperature—40 degrees or less.
- If you don't have a refrigerator thermometer, get one!

When you are ready to cook:

- Wash hands thoroughly.
- Make sure counter tops and tables are clean.
- Wash all fruits and vegetables with cold running water right before cutting or eating.
- Cook sprouts (alfalfa or bean) instead of using them raw.
- If you will be preparing meats and other foods, use two cutting boards, one for meat and one for vegetables.
- Defrost meats in the refrigerator or in the microwave, and then cook immediately.
- If you marinate meat, you must cook the leftover marinade if you plan to use it on the cooked meat.

- When grilling, use one platter and serving utensil for raw meats, and another once they are cooked.
- Do not trust your eyes and nose to accurately judge the doneness of meats. Use a meat thermometer to be safe.
- Here's how to judge when a food item is done:

Food Item	Recommended Internal Temperature or Condition
Egg dishes and casseroles	160°F
Beef, veal, pork, lamb	160°F
Poultry	180°F
Fish	Opaque flesh, flakes easily
Shellfish	Opaque throughout
Casseroles	160°F
Leftovers	Heated to 165°F
Soups, gravies	Bring to a boil
Lunch meats, hot dogs	Reheated until steaming hot
Eggs	Cooked until yolk and white are firm, not runny

If you have leftovers:

- Foods should not sit out at room temperature for longer than one hour.
- Store foods in shallow pans less than two inches deep.
- For clean up, use hot, soapy water for cutting boards and knives.

FOOD SAFETY AWAY FROM HOME

Another potential source of food poisoning problems is eating away from home. Picnics, all-day car trips, or sporting events can present problems if proper food handling techniques are not in place. The following are some tips to keep your food safe when you are on the road:

- If you are transporting food to a picnic, school, or other social event, make sure the cooler, lunchbox, or thermos is clean and dry before adding the food.
- Wrap foods well in plastic wrap or in airtight plastic containers.
- Keep cold foods cold by using a cooler, ice, and ice packs.
- Put meats on the bottom of the cooler to prevent drips onto other foods.
- Take two coolers, one for perishable foods and one for beverages.
- Pack coolers until full—they will stay colder.
- Keep the cooler in the coldest part of the car and out of the sunlight.
- If you won't have access to soap and water, bring disposable hand wipes or waterless hand-cleaning gel to clean hands before and after cooking.

If you travel to other countries, particularly in Latin America, Asia, Africa, and the Middle East, be smart and safe about the foods and beverages you consume. The following are some tips to keep you free of food-borne illnesses when you travel abroad:

- Do not drink or brush teeth with unfiltered water. Choose bottled, boiled, or sterilized water instead.
- When you buy bottled water, make sure the seal is not broken.
- Only use ice from bottled, boiled, or sterilized water. If in doubt, avoid the ice.
- Eat only fully cooked meats and fish.
- Eat only pasteurized dairy products and avoid soft cheese such as Brie, Camembert, marscapone, and cottage cheese unless they are pasteurized. You will need to ask!
- Eat only cooked vegetables.
- If you eat raw fruit, peel it yourself, and wash with clean water

before peeling. Wash hands after peeling and before eating the fruit.

- Although it may look tempting, don't buy food from street vendors.

WHEN YOU HAVE FOOD POISONING

Even with precautions, it is possible to get sick. Diarrhea is the most common symptom of food poisoning. The goal is to replace fluids and electrolytes (sodium and potassium) so you don't become dehydrated. Here are some tips to replace what your body loses:

- Start with small amounts of diluted fruit juice or undiluted sports drink, which will replace fluid and electrolytes. Try to drink four ounces every hour, or more if you can tolerate a larger volume.
- Pedialyte and Ceralyte can be used for adults and children who have diarrhea, while Infalyte can be used for infants.
- Be careful about consuming regular carbonated beverages, as the sugar content may worsen diarrhea.
- Try to avoid caffeine, which can have a laxative effect.
- Broth or bouillon can replace sodium.

As the diarrhea subsides, you may want to try to gradually introduce solid foods into your diet. Start with one item at a time, and use the following suggestions for food choices:

- Eat salty crackers or pretzels to replace sodium.
- Try foods such as oatmeal, white rice, applesauce, and bananas, which may help to slow down your bowel movements so you don't have to run to the bathroom quite so often.
- Chicken noodle or chicken rice soup with small amounts of added chicken may be easy to tolerate.
- You may want to try skinless, baked chicken with white rice, or baked potato without the skin.

- Eliminate foods such as apple juice and sugar-free candies and chewing gum. They are high in sorbitol, a sugar alcohol that can cause diarrhea and make your symptoms worse.
- Limit intake of fatty, greasy foods, which can make diarrhea worse.
- Limit intake of high-fiber foods, such as bran cereal, whole grain breads, brown rice, and fruits and vegetables, as the fiber may worsen the diarrhea.

Diarrhea can last anywhere from one day to one week. Even after the diarrhea subsides, you may have a problem with dairy products for thirty to sixty days. This is because the bacteria that causes the diarrhea can prevent the body from producing enough lactase, an enzyme the body produces to digest dairy foods.

Bottom Line

- Most food-borne illnesses can be prevented by following proper food handling techniques at home and when you travel.
- If you have any doubts about a food, throw it out!
- If you become ill after you've eaten, and are not feeling better, contact your doctor.

See appendix F for resources.

CHAPTER 5

Gastroesophageal Reflux Disease

C harlie, a very successful banker, works long hours and travels frequently. He often conducts business over late-night dinners. He began to notice an uncomfortable feeling in his chest when he went to sleep. He often woke up in the middle of the night with a burning sensation in his chest and an acid taste in his mouth. He went to the pharmacy and bought a box of antacids, but found that he needed to take more and more of them as time progressed and that the symptoms did not go away.

What Charlie suffers from is gastroesophageal reflux disease, often referred to as GERD—heartburn, indigestion, or inflammation of the walls of the esophagus. He is not alone. About 25 million Americans suffer from heartburn daily, and 60 million Americans experience heartburn once or twice a month. Twenty-five percent of pregnant women experience daily heartburn, and over half will have bouts of heartburn at some point during their pregnancy. GERD is most common in people over the age of forty, but can affect children as well.

WHAT IS GERD?

There is a valve between the esophagus and stomach called the lower esophageal sphincter (LES). When your digestive system is working well, this valve relaxes only enough to allow swallowed food to pass from the esophagus to the stomach. But if you have GERD, this valve is weakened and relaxes at the wrong time. The end result is that the acidic content of the stomach backs up into the esophagus. This acid can travel to the upper esophagus, causing a sour taste in your mouth and making you cough. This acid is very irritating to the esophagus, and can result in inflammation as well as pain.

Stomach acid surges at its greatest strength between one and three hours after meals. If you lie down after eating, there is a greater risk of acid flowing into the esophagus.

SYMPTOMS OF GERD

- Heartburn
- Acid reflux
- Difficulty swallowing (due to a narrowing of the esophagus as a result of inflammation)
- Chest pain (often worse after a heavy meal or at night)
- Chronic cough (caused by stomach acid regurgitating into the lungs)
- Hoarseness (due to acid reflux and inflammation)
- Blood in the stool or vomit (due to inflammation of the lining of the esophagus or to an esophageal ulcer)

DIAGNOSIS

There are several medical tests that can be done to diagnose GERD. If you are having symptoms, it is important to see your doctor, who may recommend one or more of the following tests: upper endoscopy, upper gastrointestinal X ray, or acid (pH) probe test.

An upper endoscopy involves placing a long, narrow tube down your throat and into your stomach and duodenum after an anesthetic is sprayed into your throat. Some people may require a light sedative. A camera attached to the tube shows areas of inflammation or damage to the esophagus.

An upper gastrointestinal X ray involves swallowing barium, a liquid that makes the lining of the esophagus and stomach more visible, before the picture is taken.

The acid (pH) probe test can help determine if you have acid reflux. The probe measures when and for how long stomach acid backs up into your esophagus. An anesthetic spray is given to numb your throat, and then a narrow tube is threaded through your nose into your esophagus. The other end of the tube is attached to a lightweight portable computer that records acid measurements over a twenty-four-hour period. This test can help your physician decide what the most effective treatment will be.

TREATMENT

It is important to treat your heartburn. The goals of treatment are to protect the esophagus from further irritation, reduce gastric acidity, and reduce the likelihood of reflux.

If you ignore the symptoms, you can end up with health problems that can be quite severe:

- Esophageal narrowing—scar tissue in the esophagus can cause food to get caught when you eat.
- Ulcer—esophageal ulcers can form as a result of excess stomach acid, and can cause bleeding, pain, and difficulty swallowing.
- Barrett's esophagus—the color of the esophageal tissue changes, so that it looks more like the tissue of the small intestine. This change can increase the risk of esophageal cancer.

Treatment for GERD consists of modifying your food choices and eating habits, and, in some cases, medications.

MEDICATIONS

Prescription or over-the-counter medications for GERD will not work if you don't make changes to other contributing factors, such as diet and eating habits. There are several products available to help with symptoms, but it is important to take the product that is most effective for you. Your doctor can determine which medication will be the best choice. The following medications are the ones most commonly used for symptom management.

- Antacids
- Prelief (calcium glycerophosphate)
- Acid blockers (Tagamet, Pepcid, Axid, Zantac)
- Proton pump inhibitors (Prevacid, Prilosec, Nexium, Aciphex, Protonix)
- Motility agents (Reglan)

Antacids are most effective in treating mild or occasional heartburn. They work by neutralizing gastric acid, and while they do provide quick relief, they do not cure the problem. Be aware that mild antacids that contain aluminum can cause constipation, whereas products with magnesium can cause diarrhea. If you take antacids, also know that the liquid form works faster than pills. Do let your physician know if you take antacids regularly.

Prelief is an over-the-counter product that neutralizes the acid in food. It is available as tablets that are taken at meal time, or as a powder that can be sprinkled on foods or in beverages. Acid blockers work by reducing acid secretion, so they can prevent acid reflux and heartburn and their effects last longer than those of antacids. These medications also help the esophagus to heal by decreasing the amount of acid that comes into contact with inflamed tissues. They are best taken before a meal. These medications are also available without a prescription, although the over-the-counter dose is not as strong as the prescription version.

Proton pump inhibitors are prescription medications that block acid production. Motility agents speed up gastric emptying, and increase the LES pressure, thereby decreasing the likelihood of reflux.

If you are taking any of these medications, do be careful with herbal preparations, as some of them can interact with GERD preparations. The following table lists potential medication and herb interactions.

Medication and Herb Interactions

Medication	Herb Interactions
Tagamet Prilosec Pepcid Axid Zantac Prevacid	Kola nut and ma huang can increase stomach acid
Tagamet Reglan Pepcid Axid Zantac	Valerian and kava can increase drowsiness
Tagamet Prilosec	Gingko, ginseng, garlic, ginger can increase the anticoagulant effect
Reglan	Ginseng, ma huang, hawthorn, saw palmetto, licorice may increase blood pressure Garlic may decrease blood pressure

SUPPLEMENTS

The nutritional supplement that may be of benefit is sodium alginate, also known as blue-green algae. It may work by neutralizing excess acid. Even though you can buy blue-green algae in a supplemental form, the purity issues of commercially available products may outweigh the benefits of its use. Sodium alginate is also an ingredient in some antacids.

It may surprise you to learn that there are certain supplements and medications that can worsen your GERD. The products that may increase symptoms of GERD are:

- Large doses of vitamin C
- Fosamax, which can cause heartburn if not taken with enough fluid, or if you lie down after taking it
- Potassium supplements
- NSAIDS (Motrin, Aleve, Advil, Nuprin, Orudis)
- Aspirin
- White willow bark
- Calcium channel blockers for high blood pressure
- Theophylline
- Certain antibiotics
- Glucosamine
- Pantethine
- Red yeast rice
- Fish oil capsules

Glucosamine may help relieve some of the pain and immobility of arthritis, but may also worsen GERD. Red yeast rice and fish oil capsules are used for the treatment of elevated cholesterol and trigylceride levels, but can worsen heartburn. If you are taking any of these products, and have noticed a worsening of your symptoms, you may want to stop taking them. Do ask your doctor about these products before you even consider using them: you may save yourself some discomfort.

THE IMPACT OF DIET

Many individuals with GERD can control their symptoms by making changes to food choices and eating habits. The combination of both offers the best chance of relieving symptoms. Unfortunately many believe they can eat whatever they want, and then just take medication. This, however, may lead to worsening of the inflammation and symptoms.

There are also several nutrition habits that people indulge in that only serve to worsen the symptoms of GERD:

- Skipping meals, then eating a lot at the next meal
- Eating the majority of calories late at night
- Eating too quickly
- Eating while rushed
- Eating a lot of high-fat foods
- Using a lot of peppermint candy or gum
- Consuming too much coffee or alcohol
- Carrying extra weight

Excess weight can be a major contributor to indigestion because of the increased pressure on the stomach and the diaphragm, a muscle that separates the chest and abdomen. This can cause the lower esophageal sphincter (LES) to relax, allowing acid to come back up. A higher Body Mass Index is associated with increased risk of GERD.

When people skip meals to avoid the discomfort of GERD, they tend to overeat at the subsequent eating time. This can distend the stomach, causing the LES to relax and increasing reflux.

Certain foods and beverages such as peppermint candy or gum, chocolate, onions, spicy foods, and alcohol relax the LES and so should be avoided. If you routinely use peppermint-flavored mints or chewing gum, you may find that your symptoms are worse. Eating a small piece of chocolate on occasion should not present a problem, but eating it on a daily basis is strongly discouraged. All types of alcohol, including beer, wine, and liquor can relax the LES. If you have heartburn, you would be wise to avoid alcohol.

Too often people assume that only acidic-tasting foods or beverages such as citrus or tomato products should be limited. While these foods *may* be irritating to the inflamed esophagus, and some individuals notice an increase in symptoms after say, drinking orange juice or eating pasta with tomato sauce, others can tolerate these foods without any problems.

Potentially Bothersome Foods or Eating Patterns

- Fatty foods
- Capsaicin, the active ingredient in cayenne pepper
- Citrus drinks and juices
- A high protein diet

Although fat-containing foods do not increase acid levels, they may increase the speed and severity of heartburn symptoms. If these foods bother you, cut down on the amount you eat and how often you eat them to see if you feel better as a result. Some people may find red pepper (cayenne) irritating, but others may not be bothered at all. Citrus drinks and juices do not cause reflux, but the acidity of these foods may stimulate sensory nerves in the inflamed esophagus, resulting in discomfort. Some individuals notice that when they switch to a very high protein diet, emphasizing meat, poultry, fish, or eggs with vegetables and little else, they may feel worse due to the increase in acid secretion produced by protein digestion.

NUTRITION SOLUTIONS

First it is important to identify which, if any, foods you find bother-some. Note these in your food diary, and mention and monitor any supplement use as well. Use the food diary to keep track of foods and symptoms. Look at the sample GERD food diary, then make copies of the blank food diary that follows. Use it to track your food triggers and symptoms. Take care to limit the amount and frequency of irritating foods and supplements. Pay attention to the times of the day when your symptoms tend to be more pronounced, and try to modify your eating patterns accordingly by changing meal size and the activities you typically do before or after meals.

Also, the following strategies can be helpful:

- Eat smaller meals.
- Eat at regularly spaced intervals.

Sample Food and Symptom Diary for GERD

Time	Food	Amount	Activities	Symptoms
7 A.M.	Toast	2 slices	reading paper	Felt okay
	Butter	2 pats		
	Orange juice	8-oz glass		
7:30 A.M.	Coffee, black	2 large mugs	1 at home, 1 in the car	A little burning
8 A.M.	Coffee, black	8-oz cup	At office desk	Acid taste in throat
9 A.M.	Water and antacid	4 gulps water	Water fountain	Burning
10 A.M.			Answering phone	Okay
12 noon	Cheeseburger	½	At restaurant	Heartburn
	Fries	10		
	Cola	12-oz glass		
12:30 P.M.	Water and antacid	8 oz water		Acid taste in mouth
1 P.M.				Better
2 P.M.	Cola	12 oz can	On the phone	A little uncomfortable
3 P.M.	Pretzels	A handful	At computer	Okay
4 P.M.				Okay
5 P.M.	Peppermint patty	2	In the car	Heartburn
6 P.M.	Pepperoni pizza	4 slices	At home watching TV	Burning in throat
6:30 P.M.	Water and antacid		Lying on sofa— home	Heartburn
7:30 P.M.			Lying on sofa	Okay
8 P.M.	2% milk	8-oz glass	On sofa	Okay
	Chocolate chip cookies	3		
9 P.M.			In bed	Burning in throat
10 P.M.	Water and antacid	4 gulps water	Watching TV news	Heartburn

Food and Symptom Diary for GERD

Time	Food	Amount	Activities	Symptoms

- Eat a lighter meal in the evening.
- Take fluids between, instead of with, meals. This can decrease the likelihood of reflux.
- Chew gum, (but not peppermint flavor) to stimulate saliva, which neutralizes stomach acid.
- Lose weight if you are overweight. Even a few pounds can make a difference.
- Make a concerted effort to relax when eating.
- Stay upright after meals. Especially do not lie down after a large lunch or dinner.
- Refrain from exercising vigorously right after eating.

On the following page is an example of a sample meal plan that may help your digestive system function more normally if you have GERD. Keep in mind that food choices, portion size, and eating habits are equally important for symptom relief.

In addition to these suggestions, here are some other behaviors and lifestyle strategies that may help to control your symptoms:

- Avoid wearing tight-fitting clothes that press on the abdomen.
- Stop smoking, as nicotine weakens the esophageal sphincter and increases acid production.
- Raise the head of your bed six to nine inches. Stacking pillows will not achieve the same effect. You can put a foam wedge under the top part of the mattress, or prop up the legs of the legs of the head of your bed with wooden blocks.
- Wait three hours after you eat before you lie down.

Bottom Line

If you don't want the pain, it is worthwhile to make some changes in your life. What you eat, when you eat, and how you eat can all affect how you feel. Medications can help your symptoms, but your food choices and eating habits may prevent the problems in the first place.

A Sample Meal Plan for GERD

Wake-Up 6 A.M.:	8-ounce glass of water
Breakfast 7 A.M.:	Cup of wheat flakes with 1% milk and a 5-inch banana
8 A.M.:	Cup of herbal tea
Midmorning Snack 10 A.M.:	3 peanut butter crackers and a tennis-ball-size serving of grapes
11 A.M.:	16-ounce bottle of water
Lunch 12:30 P.M.:	Turkey breast sandwich with lettuce, a slice of tomato and a thin spread of "light" mayonnaise;
	6 baby carrots
	handful of pretzels
1 p.m.:	10-ounce bottle of apple juice
Midafternoon Snack 3 P.M.:	A 6-ounce container of fruit-flavored yogurt and another handful of pretzels
4 P.M.:	8-ounce cup of water
Dinner 6:30 P.M.:	4-ounce baked fish filet (the size of a computer mouse);
	1 cup of frozen green beans, steamed, with no more than 1 pat of butter;
	1 cup of rice pilaf (from a boxed mix, with half the recommended butter added)
7:30 P.M.:	Cup of herbal tea
8 P.M.:	Scoop of low-fat frozen yogurt

- Determine what foods are bothersome, and how much of them you can tolerate.
- Try to eat evenly sized meals throughout the day.
- Plan your day so that you are able to finish eating several hours before lying down, or plan on having a lighter evening meal.
- Eat in a relaxed atmosphere, such as at a dinner table, instead of behind the wheel of your car or in front of a computer screen.

CHAPTER 6

Ulcers

M aria, an executive secretary for a law office, works full time, attends night school, and has two small children. Her days are pretty hectic, and most mornings find her gulping down a cup of coffee as she prepares lunch for her kids. The whole family then piles into the car. She drops the kids off at school and hurries to work, always making it to her desk just in time. She often does not eat breakfast, and works through lunch. Her boss sometimes orders in for his employees, but usually from fast food places. To help her concentrate and stay awake, especially when she has night classes, Maria drinks coffee, iced tea, and carbonated beverages with caffeine. Dinner is often very late, and quick, so that she can study or spend time with her children.

Lately, Maria has been waking up in the middle of the night with pain in her stomach, and in the morning she often feels nauseated. She tried taking antacids, but didn't feel any better. Maria made an appointment to see her doctor, who decided to do some tests. He also had the nurse give her information on a bland diet. The nurse also recommended that she see a registered dietitian to help develop a meal plan she could follow. Maria was diagnosed with a peptic ulcer, and came to see me to work on her food choices and eating habits.

WHAT ARE ULCERS?

There are two types of ulcers under the general term of peptic ulcer: *gastric* ulcer and *duodenal* ulcer. The name refers to the part of the digestive tract that is affected. A gastric ulcer occurs in the lining of the stomach. Duodenal ulcers are located in the upper part of the small intestine (duodenal). Ulcers occur when the stomach produces excess amounts of pepsin, a digestive enzyme, and acid, or when the lining of the stomach or duodenum is weak, and less able to tolerate gastric acid. Approximately one in ten Americans will develop an ulcer over the course of their lifetime.

Up to 50 percent of ulcers are caused by the bacteria Heliobacter pylori. H. pylori affects the protective coating of the stomach, causing it to become weak, and allowing acid to get through to the lining. In addition to H. pylori, here are some other factors that can contribute to ulcer formation:

- Heredity. Your risk of developing an ulcer is higher if other relatives have ulcers.
- Excessive use of nonsteroidal anti-inflammatory drugs (e.g., Motrin, Aleve, Advil).
- Cigarettes.
- Excess alcohol.
- Stress, which increases stomach acid production, and may decrease the body's ability to resist excess acid production. Stress acts more to aggravate ulcers, but does not cause ulcers to form.
- Long-term aspirin use.

SYMPTOMS

Not everyone who has an ulcer has symptoms. In some cases, though, there may be a sudden onset of pain, or nausea and vomiting. In addition, some of the symptoms of ulcers are the same as those of stomach flu. The most frequently experienced symptoms of ulcers include:

- Gnawing, burning pain in the stomach, but not a sharp pain. Sometimes this can be mistaken for hunger pangs.
- Pain that can occur between meals, typically two to three hours after meals.
- Pain in early hours of the morning, when the stomach is empty.
- Intermittent, not constant pain.
- Nausea or hunger that subsides after eating.

The following symptoms are experienced less frequently:

- Constant nausea
- Vomiting
- Loss of appetite
- Weight loss
- Back pain
- Bloating
- Burping

If you have any of the following symptoms, *contact your doctor immediately*. These symptoms could be signs of a serious problem including perforation of the stomach or duodenal wall by the ulcer, a bleeding ulcer, or obstruction of the stomach by the ulcer:

- Sharp stomach pain
- Vomiting blood
- Change in stool color, or the presence of blood in the stool

DIAGNOSIS

To learn if an ulcer is present, a physician will order an upper gastrointestinal (GI) X ray or an endoscopy.

An upper GI X ray requires swallowing barium, a liquid that makes ulcers more visible, before you have the X ray. An endoscopy involves placing a long, narrow tube down your throat and into your stomach and duodenum. A camera is attached to the tube, and if an ulcer is present, the picture will be visible on the TV monitor. Your doctor can take a sample of tissue, or biopsy, to make sure that the tissue is benign or to check for the presence of the H. pylori bacteria.

To determine if your ulcer is caused by H. pylori, the following tests are done:

- A blood test to determine whether you have H. pylori antibodies
- A breath test
- A stool antigen test

Blood tests for H. pylori can confirm the presence of the H. pylori antibodies, but cannot show if the infection is current, or if you were exposed previously. For the breath test, you blow into a plastic bag, which is then sealed. You then drink a liquid that contains radioactive carbon, which can be broken down by H. pylori. Then you blow into a second bag. If you have H. pylori, the second bag will contain the radioactive carbon as carbon dioxide. The stool antigen test checks for the presence of H. pylori in stool samples.

TREATMENT

The goals of treatment are:

- To reduce the secretion of gastric acid and pepsin
- To neutralize the gastric acid that is secreted, to decrease irritation of the lining of the stomach or duodenum
- To protect the affected area from further inflammation
- To enable the ulcerated area to heal

Medications are typically used to manage symptoms and promote healing. It is important to note that a particular eating pattern cannot cause or heal an ulcer, although it may help with symptom relief.

MEDICATIONS

- Antibiotics, if the ulcer is caused by bacteria, (Amoxicillin, Wymox, Biaxin, Flagyl, Achromycin, Prevpac, Helidac)
- Acid blockers (Zantac, Pepcid, Axid, Tagamet)
- Antacids
- Proton pump inhibitors (Prilosec, Prevacid, Nexium, Aciphex, Protonix)
- Cytoprotective agents (Carafate, Cytotec, Pepto-Bismol)

Several types of antibiotics can kill the H. pylori bacteria. Prevpac and Helidac are combination medications that contain antibiotics with a medication to suppress acid, thus protecting the lining of the stomach and small intestine. Acid blockers decrease the amount of acid secreted into the digestive tract to relieve pain and promote healing. Your physician may recommend the use of an antacid with an acid blocker, or by itself. Antacids do not reduce acid secretion, but can neutralize gastric acid and provide quick pain relief.

Proton pump inhibitors are prescription medications that block acid production. They may also inhibit H. pylori. Cytoprotective medications help to protect the lining of the stomach and small intestine. Pepto-Bismol may inhibit H. pylori activity in addition to protecting the lining of the stomach and small intestine. Carafate may cause constipation, and Cytotec can cause diarrhea. It is important to inform your doctor if you experience side effects with any of these medications.

If you are taking any of these medications, do be careful with herbal preparations. The table on the following page lists potential medication and herb interactions.

SUPPLEMENTS

Some studies have suggested that licorice root (less than 400 mg/day) may help to prevent ulcer formation. In addition, licorice root contains substances known as flavonoids, which may prevent

Medication and Herb Interactions

Medication	Herb Interactions
Tagamet Prilosec Pepcid Axid Zantac Prevacid Cytotec	Kola nut and ma huang can incréase stomach acid
Tagamet Pepcid Axid Zantac Amoxicillin Flagyl	Valerian and kava can increase drowsiness
Tagamet Prilosec Biaxin Achromycin Pepto-Bismol	Gingko, ginseng, garlic, and ginger can increase the anticoagulant effect
Pepto-Bismol	Hawthorn, ginger, garlic, ginseng, nettle can increase or decrease blood glucose

the H. pylori bacteria from forming. It is very important not to use licorice root to excess, however, as increased amounts can cause hypokalemia (low blood potassium), hyponatremia (low blood sodium), and hypertension (high blood pressure). These are caused by glycyrrhizic acid, found naturally in licorice root. So it is better to buy deglycyrrhizenated licorice, which has the glycyrrhizic acid removed—look for a licorice root product that has the letters DGL on the label. The suggested dosage for acute symptoms is one to one and half grams of DGL twenty minutes before a meal, and a chewable preparation is more effective than tablets. Make sure though, that you discuss use of this supplement with your doctor. *If you have high blood pressure or kidney problems, do not use licorice root.*

Ginger may be protective against ulcer formation, but large doses on an empty stomach may lead to ulcer formation. Some individuals notice heartburn with the use of ginger. Aloe juice may help ulcers to heal, but it can also have a laxative effect. Do check with your physician before taking either of these supplements.

IMPACT OF DIET

The process of digestion itself results in the secretion of gastric acid. And even though your diet does not cause or cure ulcers, it is very important to identify foods that you find to be irritating by using your food diary. Many people with ulcers think they have to eat a very restricted diet. That is not necessarily true, although you do need to find what you tolerate and proceed accordingly. Your food diary can be very helpful in allowing you to determine which foods are well tolerated, as well as which foods are bothersome. Be sure to record supplements as well as foods. Make copies of the food diary that follows the sample. Use it to track your food triggers and symptoms.

The following are some of the things that ulcer patients may have tried or been told to do that are incorrect:

- Assume that it is necessary to eat a bland diet.
- Eat a very restricted, unbalanced diet of just soup, cooked cereal, and gelatin to rest the stomach.
- Drink a lot of milk. (This strategy can increase stomach acid production and make ulcers worse.)
- Assume decaffeinated products are less bothersome. (Acid secretion is the same after decaffeinated as after regular beverages.)
- Eat a very high protein diet.
- Graze all day. (Your stomach secretes acid every time you eat, so if you eat too often, you may find that your symptoms are worse.)

NUTRITION SOLUTIONS

There are ways available that can help you combat any ulcers you might have. All foods are composed of the macronutrients—protein, fat, and carbohydrate—each of which has a different effect on gastric acid secretion.

Sample Food Diary for Ulcers

Time	Food	Amount	Activities	Symptoms
7 A.M.	Coffee, black	1 mug	In the car	Okay
8 A.M.	Coffee, black	2 mugs	In the office	A little burning in the stomach
9 A.M.	2% milk	8-oz glass	At my desk	Burning
9:30 A.M.	Water	4 gulps		Pain
	Antacid			
11:30 A.M.	Breaded chicken sandwich with BBQ sauce	¾	At the restaurant	A little uncomfortable
	Onion rings	5		
	Sprite	8 sips		
1 P.M.	Water	8-oz glass	Sitting at desk	Achy pain
2 P.M.	Hot tea, black	8-oz cup	At desk	Burning
3 P.M.	Saltine crackers	6	Working at desk	Better
6 P.M.	Pork chop, baked	2	At the dining room table	Okay
	Mashed potatoes	2 spoonfuls		
	Peas and carrots, frozen	½ cup		
	2% milk	12-oz glass		
7 P.M.			Watching Television	Burning
8 P.M.	Water and an antacid	8-oz glass	Watching television	A little pain
9 P.M.	Water	4-oz glass	In bed	Feeling better

Your Personal Food Diary for Ulcer Management

Time	Food	Amount	Activities	Symptoms

Nutrient	Effect on Gastric Acid Secretion
Protein	increases
Fat	decreases
Carbohydrate	has no effect

As you know, the goal for nutritional well-being and good gut health is to include a mix of protein, carbohydrate and fat. Although protein foods increase gastric acid secretion, they should not be eliminated from your diet. However, make sure that the amount of protein at each meal is only one-third of the plate. Although fat decreases gastric acid secretion, a high-fat diet may make your symptoms worse. The goal is not to eliminate fat from the diet, but to consume fat-containing foods in moderation. For overall nutritional health, try to focus on the food choices that are lower in fat. The following table lists food choices based on fat content.

High- and Lower-Fat Content Food List

Food Items	Low-Fat	High-Fat
Dairy	Skim and 1% milk, low-fat yogurt, lower-fat cheese (less than 5 grams fat per ounce)	Whole and 2% milk, cream, half-and-half, whole-milk yogurt, high-fat cheeses (more than 9 grams fat per ounce), regular sour cream
Eggs	Boiled, scrambled with minimal fat or a vegetable spray	Fried
Meats	Broiled, grilled, roasted baked, steamed, stewed; water packed canned fish	Fried meats, bacon, sausage pepperoni, salami, bologna, hot dogs
Soups	Broth, creamed with skim milk	Cream or whole-milk soups or chowders
Fat*	1 to 3 teaspoons of added oil or spread such as margarine, butter, oil, salad dressing, gravy, low-fat spreads and dressings	Mayonnaise, oil, salad dressings, gravies in amounts greater than recommended, nuts, nut butters

High- and Lower-Fat Content Food List *(continued)*

Food Items	Low-Fat	High-Fat
Snack items	Pretzels, low-fat popcorn, low-fat crackers, baked chips, rice cakes	Chips, buttery-type crackers, cheese crackers or cheese curls
Sweets	Low-fat frozen yogurt, fruit ices, sherbet, pudding made with skim milk, gelatin, vanilla wafers, gingersnaps, angelfood cake, animal crackers, reduced-fat cookies	Ice cream, doughnuts, pastries, pudding with whole milk, brownies, cookies

In addition to identifying any foods that give you trouble, there may be some other items that you find to be irritating such as spices, citrus products, and certain beverages. Before you eliminate them from your diet, keep track of how you feel when you include these items, and when you exclude them. The following items may increase gastric acid production:

- Black pepper
- Chili powder
- Mustard seed
- Nutmeg
- Citrus juices or fruits (orange, grapefruit, pineapple, lemon, tangerine)
- Sports drinks
- Cocoa
- Chocolate
- Meat extracts (gravies, bouillons)
- Coffee and tea (regular and decaffeinated)
- Alcohol

You may find that you feel better eating smaller, more frequent meals. However, this does not mean continuous eating throughout the day, which may make you feel worse. In general, the larger the meal, the greater the distention, and increase in gastric acid secretion. Eating smaller, more frequent meals may be most helpful in acute ulcers. You may also want to stop eating one hour before going to bed to see if this strategy helps with symptom relief.

Bottom Line

Managing ulcers is a combination of decreasing irritants and including items that help the inflamed areas heal. Even though what you eat can't give you an ulcer, food choices can make you feel worse or better. Be sure to do the following:

- Figure out which foods work for you and which ones give you trouble.
- Try to limit those items that can increase gastric acid secretion.
- Include a mix of nutrients at every meal.
- Try to eat regular, smaller meals throughout the day.
- Be careful of potential irritants such as smoking, alcohol, and aspirin.

CHAPTER 7

Inflammatory Bowel Diseases

J oe was a talented athlete, lettering in four sports in college. Signed by a professional baseball team in his senior year, he had plans for a rosy future. But in pre-season conditioning, he was plagued by constant diarrhea, nausea, vomiting, and fevers. The team physician told him he had the flu, and prescribed bed rest and aspirin. Joe's symptoms started to get worse, and the other team members noted that he was losing a lot of weight. He got scared when he went to the bathroom and noticed blood in the toilet, but continued to attend practice until he was so dehydrated he had to be taken by ambulance to the local hospital.

After several tests were ordered, Joe was diagnosed with Crohn's disease. He started on medications, and met with a dietitian who recommended changes in his food choices and eating schedule. Joe has resumed baseball, is playing well, and feels good overall. He has certainly learned to listen to his gut, and pay attention when he doesn't feel well.

WHAT IS INFLAMMATORY BOWEL DISEASE?

Crohn's disease and ulcerative colitis are both defined as inflammatory bowel diseases (IBD). Crohn's disease, an inflammation of all of the layers of the digestive tract, can appear anyplace, from the mouth to the anus. However, Crohn's disease occurs most commonly in the small intestine. Ulcerative colitis is an inflammation of just the inner lining of the intestinal tract and is seen in the colon (large intestine) or rectum, not in the rest of the gastrointestinal tract. These diseases occur most often in people between the ages of fifteen and thirty-five. Their causes are not known, but contributing factors include:

- The inability of the immune system to fight off an as yet unidentified virus or bacteria.
- Heredity. Inflammatory bowel diseases tend to run in families.
- Environmental factors, such as diet, stress, and inactivity.

SYMPTOMS

Symptoms for ulcerative colitis include:

- Diarrhea, which is sometimes bloody
- Abdominal pain
- Cramping

Symptoms for Crohn's disease include:

- Diarrhea, which is sometimes bloody
- Abdominal pain
- Nausea
- Vomiting
- Fever
- Weight loss
- Fatigue

In Crohn's disease, some patients can develop *fistulas,* which are abnormal connections between internal organs or between an organ and the surface of the skin. Fistulas are created from deep ulcers that penetrate through the wall of the intestine. They can lead to nutrient malabsorption, since the food leaves the intestine too rapidly for nutrients to be absorbed. They can also lead to infection. Sometimes, individuals with Crohn's disease can experience inflamed, painful, stiff, and swollen joints; skin rashes; eye inflammation; kidney stones; or gallstones.

DIAGNOSIS

Crohn's disease or ulcerative colitis can be diagnosed by the following tests:

- Blood tests to check for anemia
- Blood tests to check for a high white blood cell count, which indicates inflammation
- Stool sample to check for blood
- Upper gastrointestinal (GI) series
- Colonoscopy

For the upper GI series, you are instructed to drink a barium solution prior to X rays of your small intestine. The barium is highlighted on the X ray and can indicate areas of inflammation or abnormalities, such as narrowing, or obstruction in the intestine. The colonscopy is a test in which a long narrow tube is inserted into your rectum. This tube is attached to a computer and TV monitor, and can show areas of inflammation in the large intestine.

TREATMENT

The three goals of therapy for individuals with IBD are:

1. To control symptoms and to keep the disease in a state of remission where the need for medication is as minimal as possible
2. To be as well nourished as possible to keep the body healthy
3. To improve the quality of life

Treatment for IBD can involve surgery, medication, and nutritional solutions.

SURGICAL OPTIONS

In some cases, it is necessary for all or part of the intestines to be removed. The body still must be able to get rid of stool if the intestines are no longer available to do so. The surgeon performs a procedure called an *ostomy,* which creates an opening called the *stoma,* through which stool can leave the body. The three types of ostomy surgeries are:

- Ileostomy, in which the colon and rectum are removed
- Colostomy, in which the rectum is removed
- Ileoanal reservoir surgery, in which the individual will be able to have normal bowel movements

In an ileostomy and a colostomy, the individual will wear a bag attached to the stoma where the stool will collect. An ostomy may be a short or a permanent solution. In ulcerative colitis, removing the colon will cure the disease and newer surgical techniques can prevent the patient from needing to wear an ostomy bag. Yet this is still considered very drastic surgery, and it is not going to be the answer for everyone. Surgery for Crohn's disease patients is done to treat obstruction if the individual has strictures (intestinal narrowing), infections, or fistulas that won't heal. Surgery is *not* a cure in Crohn's disease, but when surgery is combined with medication, the chance of recurrence is lower.

MEDICATIONS

There are four basic types of medications that doctors prescribe for the treatment of IBDs:

- 5-Aminosalicylates (sulfasalazine, Asacol, Pentasa, Dipentum, Rowasa)

- Antibiotics (Flagyl, Cipro)
- Corticosteroids
- Immunosuppressants mercaptopurine (6-MP), azathioprine (Imuran), cyclosporine, methotrexate

A new medication, infliximab (Remicade) may be very helpful for patients with Crohn's disease who have fistulas.

Some of these medications can have side effects that can affect your ability and desire to eat. For example, sulfasalazine can cause nausea and diarrhea in those with sulfa allergies. Antibiotics can sometimes cause an upset stomach. Corticosteroids are very effective drugs, but can cause bone loss, and inspire a voracious appetite. In addition, corticosteroids can also cause the classic "moon face." This may be of particular concern to adolescents, who may be embarrassed about the way they look while on these drugs. If your child takes corticosteroids, and seems overly concerned about his or her appearance—to the point of wanting to stop taking medication—you may need to sit down and have a serious talk or even consider taking your child to a therapist, to discuss these issues. Imuran and 6-MP can cause nausea.

Let your doctor know immediately if you experience any of these symptoms. The medications are intended to make you feel better so you can eat well, not to prevent you from being able to eat.

Herbal supplements may interact with medications used for IBD. Check with your physician and dietitian before taking any of these.

Potential IBD Medication and Herb Interactions

Medication	Herbal Interaction
Asacol	Valerian and kava may increase drowsiness
Pentasa	
Rowasa	
Sulfasalazine	
Flagyl	
Cipro	
Corticosteroids	

Medication	Herbal Interaction
Methotrexate Dipentum	
Corticosteroids Cyclosporine Dipentum Methotrexate	Ginseng, ma huang, hawthorn, saw palmetto, licorice root may increase blood pressure Garlic may decrease blood pressure
Azathioprine Corticosteroids Cyclosporine Dipentum Flagyl Methotrexate 6-MP Sulfasalazine	Gingko, garlic, ginger, ginseng may increase the anticoagulant effect
Cipro Methotrexate Sulfasalazine	St. John's Wort may increase photosensitivity
Corticosteroids Cyclosporine	Hawthorn, ginger, garlic, nettle may increase or decrease blood glucose

THE IMPACT OF DIET

Good nutrition is vital to maintaining a healthy body and to prevent nutritional deficiencies, which can make you feel worse. But there is no clear association between what one eats and how it affects IBD. Too often, someone may feel guilty about eating a "bad" food that caused the illness. Not true! Diet is *not* the cause of inflammatory bowel diseases. Still, some people find that certain foods are not well tolerated or may trigger symptoms such as diarrhea, nausea, or vomiting.

Patients often try to adopt the following unwise eating strategies in an attempt to reverse or prevent IBD:

- *Eating all or nothing of a certain food.* Often, a person who is feeling well will try to cram in lots of a favorite food, thinking that this good feeling may not last long, so why not take advantage of it. Although a varied diet is certainly the goal, feast-or-famine eating patterns can cause gastrointestinal symptoms such as stomach upset, abdominal pain, nausea, or gas. Gradual changes in eating can keep symptoms to a minimum while expanding food choices to the maximum.

- *Eliminating entire food groups.* Very often, people with IBDs take all dairy products out of the diet. Unless someone has lactose intolerance, where the body cannot break down lactose, this type of restriction is unnecessary. It is comforting to know that most people with IBD are not lactose intolerant.

- *Relying on supplements instead of food.* Although these products are often sold for symptom relief, herbal, vitamin, and mineral supplements are not a source of calories and cannot serve as a substitute for food. Certainly a multivitamin-mineral supplement can help ensure you are meeting your daily requirements, but only in addition to food, not as a replacement for meals.

- *Erratic eating patterns.* Many people with IBDs eat infrequently, and without consistency. Establishing regular eating episodes can contribute to digestive comfort, as well as helping to improve your nutritional well-being.

- *Fad diets designed to treat IBD.* Avoid the fad diets, and supplements geared to people with IBDs. No single food can cause IBD, or put the body into remission. Some of these diets are very restrictive, which can cause more problems for a person who already may not be eating well. Others recommend a slew of herbal and other supplements, which may be more irritating than soothing to the gut. Follow the advice, "if it sounds too good to be true, it probably is."

- *Not eating enough food over all.* Not eating may seem logical, especially if you notice pain, bloating, and other symptoms after meals. The problem is that depriving your body of necessary fuel and nutrients will actually make you weaker and sicker than trying to eat.

From a nutritional standpoint, IBDs can contribute to malnutrition in the following ways:

- Limited food intake due to pain in the digestive tract after eating
- Increased nutrient requirements when the body is in a state of inflammation
- Decreased absorption of nutrients when the digestive tract is inflamed
- Loss of nutrients, particularly protein, vitamins, and minerals when these diseases are active
- Weight loss, which affects energy levels and the ability to carry out daily activities

So how do you manage IBD through proper nutrition? No single suggested diet or eating pattern is going to work for everyone with IBD. Yet the goal is the same: to achieve a state of eating and lifestyle that is as healthy and inclusive as possible, one that can be flexible enough to be modified depending on how you feel. In fact, eating can vary from day to day. On the days you feel terrific you may be able to tolerate a variety of foods. On other days, you may notice that most items are bothersome, even though they were perfectly fine the day before. Don't worry about this; concentrate on the positive, and follow the upcoming suggestions. Remember, any food is better for the body than none at all.

NUTRITION SOLUTIONS FOR INFLAMMATORY BOWEL DISEASES

Sally was diagnosed with Crohn's disease about two years ago. She had been overweight, and was absolutely ecstatic when she started to notice that she was losing weight rapidly, without dieting. The honeymoon was short-lived, however, as constant trips to the bathroom were leaving her weak, tired, and unable to get through her work day efficiently. When she came to see me, the first thing she told me was that she felt like she "rents food." This is a very accurate description; as she was going to the bathroom ten to twenty times most days, food hardly had time to stick around in her system!

What Sally described is not unusual for individuals with Crohn's disease and ulcerative colitis, but she, like others, was very confused as to where to start to change her diet.

A good place to start is with a food diary, which can help you to identify bothersome foods and eating behaviors. To help determine what foods and eating habits may be causing symptoms, you should keep a diary of all foods and beverages consumed, as well as the amount. Record the time, any activities while eating, and symptoms. You should also record any supplements you use regularly. Make copies of the food diary that follows the sample. Use it to track your food triggers and symptoms.

After filling out your food diary and noticing what seems to bother you, select no more than one to two nutrition goals for yourself, such as increasing fruit and vegetable intake, or eating a greater variety of foods. Then monitor any progress, or reduction of symptoms. For example, note when you experience improved energy, less frequent trips to the bathroom, or less abdominal pain.

Most individuals with IBD are able to identify foods that seem to be better tolerated. Many people find their IBD goes into remission, then, with medications, diet changes, and changes in lifestyle. In these individuals, food choices can be quite varied, and without restrictions. However, there may be times when symptoms are severe and you may be physically unable to eat. In these instances, an IV may be needed to deliver nutrients.

For now, let's identify those foods and supplements that may be bothersome to the majority of those with Crohn's disease or ulcerative colitis.

FOODS AND SUPPLEMENTS THAT MAY BE BOTHERSOME

These foods may be particularly bothersome so you may want to avoid them:

- Foods with excessive fat, such as French fries, bacon, pepperoni, and fried chicken

Sample Food and IBD Symptom Diary

Time	Food	Amount	Activities	Symptoms
7 A.M.	Cornflakes	1 cup	At the kitchen table	Felt okay
	2% milk	4 ounces		
	Apple juice	6-oz glass		
8 A.M.	Tea, black, plain	10-oz mug	In the car	Upset stomach
9 A.M.	Tea, black, plain and a multivitamin-mineral supplement and ginseng	8-oz cup	At office desk	Feel need to go to the bathroom
9:05 A.M.			Rushing to bathroom	Diarrhea
10 A.M.	Water	10-oz glass	At desk	A little queasy
12 noon	Chicken-rice soup	A bowl	At desk	Feel churning in stomach
	Ritz crackers	4		
	Applesauce	4-oz container		
	Ginger ale	½ of 12-oz can		
12:30 P.M.				Abdominal cramping
1 P.M.	Tea	8-oz cup		Okay
3 P.M.	Ritz crackers	4		Okay
5 P.M.	Ginger ale	Other half of can		A little rumbling
6:30 P.M.	Scrambled eggs, no fat added	2	At home	A little queasy
	White toast, dry	1 slice		
	2% milk	8-oz glass		
8 P.M.	Gelatin and a Vitamin C tablet and gingko	½ cup	Watching TV	Okay

Your Personal Food and IBD Symptom Diary

Time	Food	Amount	Activities	Symptoms

- Caffeine-containing beverages (coffee, tea, and soda), which can have a laxative effect
- Caffeine-containing herbs (guarana, mate, kola nut), which can have a laxative effect
- Alcohol, which can cause gastrointestinal upset
- Acidic foods and beverages (citrus fruits and juices, tomato products), which can cause gastrointestinal distress
- High-fiber foods (bran cereals, fruits and vegetables, dried beans)

As to supplements that may be bothersome, there are several products, even ones designed specifically for colon health. But some can even *cause* digestive difficulties. You may need to be careful when taking the following products, and always let your health care professional know what you are taking.

Products	*Gastrointestinal Side Effects*
Bone meal Calcium Fructo-Oligosaccharides	Abdominal bloating
Iron	Abdominal pain/bloating
Psyllium husk	Abdominal distention
Chitosan Fish oil capsules Flaxseed oil Glucosamine	Diarrhea
Glucosamine/chondroitin Iron	Nausea

FOODS TO CHOOSE

Since the goal is variety and balance with your food choices, and since there is not one food that can meet all your nutritional needs, each meal should include a *mix* of nutrients, or at least one food item from each column in the following table at every meal and snack. To be as sensitive to the workings of your digestive system as possible, it is better to start with a small amount of the food in question. A half-cup serving of fruits or vegetables may be too hard to tolerate, but a tablespoon may work nicely. Customize your portion size to meet *your* needs and comfort level. Also, make sure to include a beverage at every meal and snack, so you will be well hydrated.

Carbohydrate	*Protein*	*Fat*
Bread	Lean beef	Butter
Whole grain bread	Pork loin/chop	Margarine
White rice	Veal	Mayonnaise
Brown rice	Lamb	Salad dressings
Pasta	Chicken, skinless	Sour cream
Cereals	Fish (fresh,canned)	Oils
Whole grain cereals	Shellfish	Bacon
Crackers	Cheese	Olives
Fruits	Cottage cheese	Nuts
Vegetables	Eggs	Nut butters
Fruit juices	Soy products	
Soda	Milk	
Milk	Dried beans/peas	
Candy	Yogurt	
Cookies		
Cake/pastries		
Ice cream/frozen yogurt		
Yogurt		
Waffles/pancakes		

Individuals with chronic diarrhea may decrease the frequency of bowel movements by limiting intake of high-fiber foods such as bran cereals, brown rice, fruits and vegetables. It may help if you choose well-cooked vegetables; canned or cooked fruits without skins; and white breads instead of whole grain products. Those with strictures (narrowing) in the intestine may benefit from limiting intake of fruit and vegetable skins, popcorn, seeds, and bran cereals, as these foods can get caught in the narrowed areas, and increase the risk of bowel obstruction. Read the nutrition facts panel on food labels and use the dietary fiber information as your guide to selecting products with the least amount of fiber. The goal is not to eliminate fruits and vegetables entirely, but to experiment to find a comfort level.

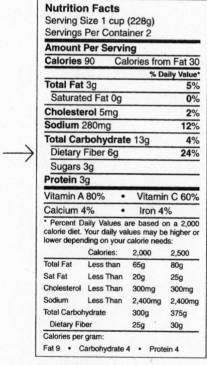

Source: FDA and CFSAN

Figure 7.1–Food label highlighting dietary fiber

If you find that fat-containing foods can be bothersome, use your food diary to determine what type and how much fat you can tolerate in your diet.

EATING HABITS TO FOLLOW

To encourage better tolerance to foods, try to do the following:

- Relax before, during, and after meals by listening to soothing music, engaging in enjoyable discussion of things that interest you, or eating in a pleasant place.
- If you eat at work, try to unplug the phone, turn off the computer, or eat away from your desk.
- Make eating purposeful; try not to be distracted when you eat.
- When you are finished eating, sit for a few minutes and relax.
- Eat at regular intervals, every three or four hours, instead of taking large, infrequent meals.
- Take small bites and chew food well.
- Sip beverages; don't gulp.

When you are experiencing symptoms, such as abdominal pain, nausea, vomiting, diarrhea, or fever, food choices may need to be limited until symptoms subside. Do not choose to continue to eat a very restrictive diet whether or not you are experiencing symptoms. This can lead to a very unbalanced, nutrient-poor eating pattern that can leave you feeling tired, weak, and unable to get through a day.

SPECIFIC RECOMMENDATIONS FOR ULCERATIVE COLITIS

Ideally, if you have ulcerative colitis and are symptom-free, you don't have to restrict anything in your diet. But if you are experiencing abdominal pain and diarrhea, you may want to limit the following foods until your symptoms subside.

- High-fiber foods: fruits and vegetables (including skins), bran cereals or breads, dried beans, and peas
- Caffeine in beverages and herbal supplements
- Concentrated sweets, including fruit juices, fruit drinks, and candies, which can contribute to diarrhea
- Alcohol, which can be irritating to the digestive tract
- Sugar alcohols (sorbitol, mannitol, xylitol), often found in sugarless gums, candies, and over-the-counter medications, which can cause diarrhea in certain individuals

Limit these foods by downsizing the portions of foods you normally eat, or substituting another form of the food. For example, if you are experiencing diarrhea, and are trying to cut back on fruits and vegetables, cut the portion size in half, and aim for only one serving per meal—either fruit or vegetable, not both together. Sometimes, canned fruit in light syrup, or canned vegetables are easier to tolerate than fresh. Peeled fruit can also be easier to tolerate than the whole fruit.

As your symptoms subside, add foods back gradually by slightly increasing the portion, so that you can determine what feels comfortable for you.

SUPPLEMENTS TO TRY FOR ULCERATIVE COLITIS

If you are taking Sulfasalazine, it is a good idea to take a daily folate supplement of 400 IU. A multivitamin-mineral supplement with iron is indicated, especially if you have experienced blood in your bowel movements. You don't have to buy a high-cost or high-potency product; just aim for one that has vitamins and minerals, an expiration date, and the USP symbol, which indicates the product's ability to be absorbed well. Take supplements *with* food, not in place of food, and never exceed the dosage on the bottle. More is always worse, not better, for the body.

Research suggest that psyllium seed may help those with ulcerative colitis by encouraging the growth of benefical bacteria in the

Nutrition Solutions during Ostomy

- Eat smaller, more frequent meals.

- Add in new foods one at a time.

- Be sure to drink enough fluid so you don't get dehydrated. Ideally drink a minimum of eight glasses of fluid a day.

- Refer to chapter 12 for information on how to decrease gas.

- Refer to chapter 14 for information on how to prevent diarrhea.

- Refer to chapter 15 for information on how to prevent constipation.

- Since odor is a concern with an ostomy, you may want to limit the following foods that can cause odor:

  Fish

  Coffee

  Onions or garlic

  Asparagus

  Eggs

  Poultry

- The following foods may actually reduce the odor of your stool:

  Cranberry juice

  Buttermilk (Do not use these if you are lactose intolerant.)

  Yogurt (Do not use these if you are lactose intolerant.)

  Parsley

  Spearmint

colon. Psyllium may also increase the production of butyrate, a fatty acid with anti-inflammatory action. The dose of psyllium seed is twenty grams per day. It can be mixed in juice or water.

Omega-3 fatty acid (fish oil) supplements may be beneficial for those with ulcerative colitis because of its anti-inflammatory effect. Before you try these, be aware that fish oil capsules sometimes can cause stomach upset, heartburn, or a bad taste in the mouth. Check with your physician before self-medicating with fish oil supplements. If you can tolerate fish, you may want to try to increase your intake of fatty fish, and aim to include salmon, mackerel, herring, and sardines, in small amounts (3-ounce serving) several times a week.

If you have had surgery for ulcerative colitis, you may want to try the dietary strategies on the preceding page to make it easier to manage your ostomy.

SPECIFIC RECOMMENDATIONS FOR CROHN'S DISEASE

The goal is to eat as varied and inclusive a diet as possible, but if you have fat malabsorption, or strictures (narrowing) in the colon, it may be necessary to be more restrictive and selective with food choices. In general, the recommendations for Crohn's disease are:

- Smaller, more frequent meals, which can help to prevent the discomfort associated with a large volume of food in the gut at one time, and can also help to keep energy levels up by fueling the body more frequently.
- When symptoms are present, it is a good idea to limit high-fiber foods (fruits, vegetables, bran cereals or bread, whole grains, dried beans and peas).
- If you have strictures in the intestine, stay away from beans, nuts, seeds, or kernels.
- Avoid popcorn, peas, and corn, which can become stuck, or can be irritating to the intestine.

- If you are lactose-intolerant, try to limit lactose-containing foods and beverages in your regular diet.
- If you have fat malabsorption, limiting fat intake can be helpful. You can do this by:

  Broiling, grilling, or baking meats

  Cooking without adding extra butter or margarine

  Choosing low- or nonfat dairy products

  Choosing low- or nonfat snack items, cookies, frozen desserts

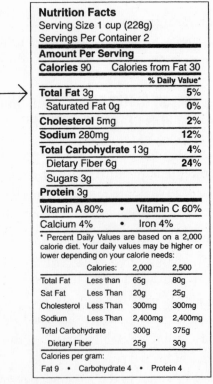

Source: FDA and CFSAN

Figure 7.2—Food label highlighting total fat

Preparing foods without added sauces or gravies

Limiting margarine, butter, mayonnaise, and salad dressings, or using low-fat or nonfat products

Read the nutrition facts panel on food labels and use the total fat information as your guide for selecting lower-fat items.

- If you have fat malabsorption, you may also need to watch your intake of oxalate-containing foods, which can contribute to kidney stones. If you have been told to limit oxalate-containing foods, try not to eat or drink:

Rhubarb

Nuts or nut butters

Chocolate

Teas

Draft beer

- If you experience short bowel syndrome as a result of Crohn's disease, see the end of this chapter for specific recommendations.

SUPPLEMENTS TO TRY FOR CROHN'S DISEASE

Since eating can sometimes be difficult with Crohn's disease, a multi-vitamin-mineral supplement can provide the micronutrients that are sometimes limited when the diet is restricted. Eating food is still important, however, as the supplements do not provide fuel to the body. Sometimes, though, eating meals can be impossible, especially with a flare-up, or an increase in symptoms. If eating is difficult, it is a good idea to keep a few meal replacement products on hand to provide a quick, easy, well-tolerated food when you don't feel like eating. Here is a list of commercially available products:

Higher Fat	*Clear Liquid*	*Modified fat*
Boost (contains lactose)	EnLive!	Lipisorb
Ensure	Subdue	Peptamen
Resource		Modulen

Carnation Instant Breakfast (contains lactose)

Whether you have Crohn's disease or Ulcerative Colitis, you may also find it helpful to follow the following sample menu plan if you are experiencing a flare-up.

Sample Menu to Follow during Flare-ups

Breakfast: A poached egg with a slice of Italian toast, and a little fruit spread if desired, but without added butter or margarine

decaffeinated tea

Midmorning: ½ cup canned peaches mixed with ½ cup Cream of Wheat (prepared with water)

8 ounces of water to drink

Lunch: Chicken noodle soup with extra chicken added (either a plain, baked chicken breast, or canned chicken breast);

a few Saltine crackers

Midafternoon: ½ turkey sandwich

½ cup applesauce

a cup of herbal (noncaffeinated) tea with a splash of cranberry juice added

Dinner: 4-ounce piece of baked fish, with a few breadcrumbs, 1 teaspoon light margarine, and a splash of lemon, if desired

½ cup cooked rice in chicken or vegetable broth

½ cup steamed green beans, without added fat

8 ounces of low-fat milk, if tolerated, or diluted juice (half water, half juice)

Evening Snack: Frozen fruit bar or Popsicle

SHORT BOWEL SYNDROME

Short bowel syndrome occurs either when the small bowel cannot function because of disease, or when it has been surgically removed. Some individuals with Crohn's disease develop regional enteritis, which destroys the functioning of the ileum. If more than 30 percent of the intestine is removed, symptoms will occur. Symptoms of short bowel syndrome can include:

- Weight loss
- Diarrhea
- Abdominal bloating
- Cramping
- Heartburn
- Fatigue
- Weakness
- Food sensitivities
- Steatorrhea, or fat in the stools
- Stunted growth in children

Some individuals with short bowel syndrome will require specialized nutrition support. Determining factors include:

- Length of the remaining colon
- Site of the resection
- Condition of the remaining bowel
- Adaptation of the remaining small bowel
- Presence of the ileocecal valve

Up to one-half of the small bowel can be removed without the patient experiencing much difficulty from a nutrition perspective. If the jejunum, or middle part of the small bowel is removed, lactose intolerance will result. If the ileum, or final portion of the small bowel is removed, fat malabsorption and vitamin B_{12} deficiency are more likely to occur. The small bowel is remarkably adaptable, and after resection, the remaining small intestine will increase absorptive surface area and slow down transit time to allow for a greater percentage of nutrients to be absorbed.

Individuals with short bowel syndrome are at increased risk for malnutrition especially when the majority of the small intestine is removed, because the remaining bowel cannot absorb adequate nutrients, water, vitamins, and minerals. The ileocecal valve, which separates the small intestine from the colon, slows down the emptying of food into the colon, so if this valve is removed, diarrhea may result. The ileocecal valve also prevents waste in the colon from returning to the small bowel. One of the waste products is bacteria, and if the valve is no longer present, bacteria can enter the small intestine, resulting in more diarrhea.

If you have short bowel syndrome, it is very important to find a dietitian to help you develop a meal plan you can live with. Call your local hospital, or log onto the American Dietetic Association's web site, www.eatright.org, and follow the link to "Find a Dietitian."

The goals of nutritional management of short bowel syndrome are to:

- Prevent malnutrition
- Prevent dehydration
- Encourage intestinal adaptation to increase nutrient absorption by increasing the size of the remaining gut, and increasing the time that nutrients remain in contact with the intestinal mucosa

NUTRITION SOLUTIONS

Although you will want to meet with a registered dietitian to develop an individualized meal plan, the following table lists general recommendations for diet for short bowel syndrome.

Food List for Short Bowel Syndrome

Choose more	Limit

Fluids

Sports drink	Fruit juice
Sugar-free beverages	Regular soda
Diet soda	Sweetened tea or coffee
Artificially sweetened tea	Water

Carbohydrate-containing foods

Rice	Cookies
Pasta	Cakes
Bread	Pies
Unsweetened hot or cold cereals	Sweetened cereals
Potatoes	Sugar
Bagels	Honey
English muffins	Syrup
Pretzels	Jelly/jams
Crackers	Sherbet, ice cream
	Fruit or juice (no more than one serving per meal)

Protein-containing foods

Fish, canned fish in water	Fried fish, canned fish in oil
Lean beef, tenderloin, chuck	"Prime" cuts, regular ground beef
Extra lean ground beef	
Pork	Ribs
Ham	Bologna, sausage, pepperoni, bacon, frankfurters
Eggs, egg substitutes	
Skinless poultry	Poultry with skin, duck
Low-fat cheese (less than 5 grams fat per serving), or soy cheese if you are lactose intolerant	High-fat cheese (more than 9 grams fat per serving)
Low-fat cottage cheese	Regular cottage cheese
Low-fat yogurt	Regular yogurt
Skim milk	Whole milk, or if you are lactose intolerant, you may need to use Lactaid milk or lactase enzymes (See chapter 11 for more information)
Tofu	
Dried beans	
Peanut butter (higher in fat, so you may have to experiment with amounts to determine your tolerance)	

(continued)

Food List for Short Bowel Syndrome *(continued)*

Choose more	Limit
Fat-containing foods	
Fat-free mayonnaise, salad dressings, vegetable spray, fat-free margarine	No more than 1 tablespoon per day of butter, margarine, oil, salad dressing, mayonnaise, cream cheese, nuts, nut butter

For individuals with short bowel syndrome, six small meals throughout the day are recommended, rather than three large ones, and four ounces of fluid should be taken at each eating episode.

Bottom Line

If you have an inflammatory bowel disease, try to do the following:

- Pay attention to what you eat.
- Figure out what foods and portion sizes work best for you.
- Keep a few supplements on hand for days when it is too difficult to eat.
- Focus on what you *can* have and make those foods a regular part of your eating plan.

CHAPTER 8

Irritable Bowel Syndrome

I magine waking up, getting out of bed ready to start the day, and having to make a mad dash for the bathroom. This scenario was a daily occurrence for Naomi, who would have to go to the bathroom several times before leaving for work. And she would never eat anything before she left her house for fear of not being able to make it to the office without having an accident. She didn't want to tell her doctor, because when she had mentioned this to her previous physician, she was told it was all in her head and that if she would relax, she would be just fine.

Naomi's symptoms are real. Unfortunately, all too often patients with irritable bowel syndrome are told that they aren't physically sick. Many with this condition suffer silently, assuming that there is no treatment, and that they will just have to learn to live with it.

WHAT IS IRRITABLE BOWEL SYNDROME?

Irritable bowel syndrome, or IBS, is very common, affecting 1 out of 10 individuals, or 22 million Americans annually. Approximately 70 percent of those with IBS are women. This is the most frequently diagnosed digestive disorder. IBS is a functional bowel disorder,

99

meaning that the results of an X ray, colonoscopy, or sigmoidoscopy come back normal. Just as the name implies, functional bowel disorder is one where there is a problem with the workings of the gut.

SYMPTOMS

The symptoms of IBS can include any of the following:

- Lower abdominal pain
- Constipation
- Diarrhea
- Alternating constipation and diarrhea
- Bloating
- Mucus in the stools

Some people say that they feel as if they still need to go to the bathroom, even when they have just gone. Others experience chest discomfort and excessive gas. Others complain of fatigue, headaches, and urinary problems. There is no cure for IBS, but patients can learn how to manage symptoms.

DIAGNOSIS

A positive diagnosis is based on criteria that include:

- Abdominal pain that is relieved after going to the bathroom
- Changes in stool frequency
- Changes in stool appearance
- A feeling of incomplete evacuation
- Passage of mucus

There are two types of IBS diagnosed in children: diarrhea-predominant IBS and pain-predominant IBS. Diarrhea-predominant IBS is more common in very young children under age three. Pain-predominant IBS, which appears more often in children from ages six to eighteen, poses more of a concern, since eating aggravates the pain. A child who is in pain may choose to eat less to feel better, resulting in weight loss and potential nutrient deficiencies.

SYMPTOM TRIGGERS

In general, people with IBS have a very sensitive gastrointestinal tract that causes symptoms to occur in response to certain triggers, including:

- Stress, particularly emotional stress
- Activity
- Diet
- Hormonal changes

Stress

Stress can affect the digestive tract even in someone with a well-functioning gut, but individuals with IBS tend to have an overactive or hyperresponsive stress response. Many have experienced significant life stressors such as physical or sexual abuse, divorce, or death of a loved one. Learning relaxation and stress management techniques, such as deep breathing, meditation, or visualization, can be very helpful in decreasing the intestinal reaction to stress and providing symptom relief.

Activity

Some people with IBS find that physical activity can cause symptoms. A person who has frequent bouts of diarrhea may find that jogging or aerobics leads to a dash to the toilet (probably not the destination the jogger had in mind). The answer may be to find an exercise that is more gut-friendly, such as swimming, Pilates, or strength training.

Diet

Shirley, a patient of mine, came into my office complaining that she was "sick" of eating. Every time she ate she experienced heartburn, nausea, abdominal pain, and diarrhea. Shirley said it wasn't worth it to eat anymore, and wanted to know if there was a pill she could take to replace food.

Shirley was experiencing an adverse food reaction. In those with IBS, these reactions can include:

- Nausea
- Vomiting
- Indigestion
- Bloating
- Diarrhea
- Abdominal pain
- Constipation

Since one of the triggers for IBS symptoms is eating, many people with IBS make drastic changes in food choices or meal size and frequency in an attempt to help with symptoms. When we eat, the stomach stretches and releases hormones, which prepare the intestine for food digestion. For those with IBS, a few bites of food can cause the bowel to react, leading to pain or a need to rush to the bathroom.

Hormonal Changes

Women who have IBS may notice that their symptoms are worse around the time of the menstrual cycle. This is caused by an increase of estrogen and progesterone, as well as the production of prostaglandins. Estrogen can slow gastric emptying, resulting in a decrease in gastrointestinal motility and transit. The net effect is an increase in bloating, pain, and constipation. Fluctuations in progesterone can also worsen symptoms. At the time of menses, the body secretes substances called prostaglandins, which affect muscle contractions in the colon and can lead to an increase in abdominal cramps and diarrhea.

TREATMENT

Surgery is not an option for those with IBS. Symptom relief is the goal, as well as achieving and maintaining good nutritional health. Treatment needs to be individualized, but typically consists of one or more of the following:

- Medications
- Changes in diet and eating habits
- Pain management
- Supplements

Medications may be prescribed that help with symptoms, but what, when, and how you eat remain very important ways to achieve good gut health. Learning pain management techniques such as deep breathing, hypnotherapy, or visualization, also can help

---

The Latest Findings on IBS

Studies have shown that the digestive pain associated with IBS is from an increased nerve sensitivity, rather than from spasms of the intestinal muscles. In other words, people with IBS may have a heightened sensitivity to pain, causing them to feel more uncomfortable. Research has also shown that the brains of IBS patients may not be able to produce substances that block the feeling of pain that occurs in response to the bowel stretching as they eat.

Recent research also has demonstrated that some individuals with IBS may have more bacteria than usual in the small intestine, which may be treated by antibiotics.

improve your quality of life. If you choose to use vitamin-mineral or herbal supplements, be aware that they are not a replacement for good eating, stress management, and physical activity.

If you have a young child with IBS, you should encourage your child to train his or her bowels to empty at regular, specified times during the day to establish a routine.

MEDICATIONS

The medications prescribed for IBS depend on the symptoms experienced, but here are some of the commonly prescribed medications:

For pain: Antispasmodics, including Bentyl, Levsin, or Robinol, which are taken before a meal to decrease the reactivity of the bowel.

For diarrhea: Loperamide (Imodium), Cholestyramine, Bismuth (Pepto-Bismol).

For constipation: Fiber, osmotic laxatives such as milk of magnesia or Lactulose, stool softeners (Colace, Surfak).

To decrease intestinal sensitivity: Tricyclic antidepressants, including Imipramine, Elavil, and Anafranil (pain relief can take up to four to six weeks with these medications), selective serotonin re-uptake inhibitors such as Zoloft and Prozac.

If you are taking any herbal supplements, or are considering doing so, and you are on medication for IBS symptoms, it is important to let your doctor know first. Certain herbs can interact with medications. The table on the following page lists the medications used for IBS and potential herbal interactions.

THE IMPACT OF DIET

Unfortunately, there is no "irritable bowel syndrome diet." As with other digestive disorders, when you are in pain, you are going to try to eliminate the item that causes you discomfort. With IBS, food can often cause the symptoms. Too often, people with IBS try to make

Potential Herbal and IBS Medication Interactions

Medication	Herbal Interaction
Anafranil Bentyl Cholestyramine Elavil Imipramine Imodium (Loperamide) Prozac Zoloft	Valerian and kava can increase drowsiness
Bismuth Colace Elavil Imipramine	Hawthorn, ginger, garlic, ginseng, and nettle can increase or decrease blood glucose
Anafranil Elavil	Ginseng, hawthorn, ephedra (ma huang), saw palmetto, and licorice may increase blood pressure
Imipramine Zoloft	Garlic may decrease blood pressure
Bismuth Cholestyramine Zoloft	Gingko, garlic, ginger, and ginseng increase the anticoagulant effect
Imipramine Elavil Anafranil Prozac	St. John's Wort can exacerbate the effect of the medication
Anafranil Prozac Zoloft	Yohimbe can increase anxiety and decrease the effectiveness of the medication

drastic changes in their diet to improve symptoms, with some unpleasant consequences. Here are four strategies you may want to *avoid*:

1. *Eliminating meals.* Not eating is not good for your gut or the rest of your body, and can result in decreased energy, weight loss, and fatigue.
2. *Avoiding entire food groups.* Eliminating all fruits and vegetables, or all grain products leads to a very unbalanced and monotonous diet.

3. *Adding too much fiber.* Fiber may be helpful if you suffer from constipation, but adding too much too soon will make your gut feel worse, not better.
4. *Eating while rushed.* Since stress is a trigger for IBS, don't try to eat a meal when you are upset or in a hurry. You may have an increase in your symptoms if you eat on the run, or in response to stress.

Some food items may cause discomfort for you, so it is very important to keep a food diary so that you can start to identify foods that may give you trouble. The following is an example of a food and symptom diary. Make copies of the food diary that follows the sample and plan on keeping the food diary for several days to try to establish a pattern. Remember to record any supplements you take, such as vitamins, minerals, herbs, sports bars, or any other products. Sometimes, it may be the supplements that are being poorly tolerated, and not just the food.

NUTRITION SOLUTIONS

The following foods are the ones that tend to be most bothersome to those with IBS. See how many of them you eat regularly. You may want to try to cut back on these foods one at a time, to see if you have fewer symptoms.

Potentially Bothersome Foods

Fried foods.

Dried beans.

Caffeine (coffee, tea, colas, herbs such as guarana, maté, and kola nut).

Carbonated beverages.

Alcohol.

Sample Food, Supplement, and IBS Symptom Diary

Time	Food/ Supplement	Amount	Activities	Symptoms
7 A.M.	Cheerios	1 cup	Standing at the sink	Felt okay
	2% milk	4 oz		
	Banana	½ of 5-inch		
8 A.M.	Tea, black, plain Calcium tablets	10-oz mug 2 (500 mg each)	In the car	Rumbling
9 A.M.			At office desk	Gassy
9:15 A.M.			Rushing to bathroom	Diarrhea
10 A.M.	Apple juice	10-oz bottle	At desk	A little queasy
10:30 A.M.			Bathroom	Diarrhea
12 noon	Turkey sandwich	4 bites	At the computer	Uncomfortable
	Herbal tea	8-oz cup		
2 P.M.	Tea, black, plain	12-oz mug	Relaxing at desk	Better
3 P.M.	Applesauce, sweetened	4-oz carton	Working at desk	Okay
4 P.M.	Ginger ale	½ of can	On the phone	Bloated
5 P.M.			Driving home	Gassy
5:30 P.M.			Lying on sofa	Bloated
6 P.M.	Chicken breast, skinless, baked, fat-free dressing	Palm-size	At the dining room table	Okay
	White rice, plain	½ cup		
	Green beans, canned, plain	2 Tbsp.		
	Lemonade, from powder	8-oz glass		
7 P.M.			Watching TV news	Okay
8 P.M.	Fruit ice	½ cup	Paying bills	A little abdominal pain
9 P.M.	Water	4-oz glass	In bed	Feeling better

Personal Food, Supplement, and IBS Symptom Diary

Time	Food/ Supplement	Amount	Activities	Symptoms

Cabbage family vegetables (broccoli, cauliflower, cabbage, brussels sprouts).

Sugar alcohols (sorbitol, mannitol in sugar-free products, apple juice, and some liquid medications). Check the label of your medications for the presence of sugar alcohols such as sorbitol, mannitol, and xylitol.

Fructose (in fruits and fruit juices).

Lactose (in dairy products).

Some people with IBS notice that symptoms are worse after eating fatty or fried foods. This is because fat causes the muscles of the large intestine to contract, resulting in pain. Also, chewing a lot of sugar-free gum, or eating sugar-free mints, can cause abdominal cramping, bloating, and diarrhea due to the presence of the artificial sweetener sorbitol. If you notice that dairy products cause trouble, you may have lactose intolerance, not IBS.

Beans and cabbage family foods may cause more gas and bloating. Alcohol and caffeine can stimulate the intestines, resulting in more frequent bowel movements. *(For additional information on dietary recommendations for bloating, gas, lactose intolerance, constipation, and diarrhea, refer to those specific chapters.)*

The goal for sufferers of IBS is not to eliminate all of the foods just listed. However, you may want to pick the ones you eat most frequently, remove it from your diet for two weeks, and see if you notice a difference in symptoms. Then reintroduce the food and see what happens. Remember, only experiment with *one food at a time*. If you are going through a particularly stressful time at work or at home, don't pick that time to start changing your diet. Wait until life settles down a little so you can get a better idea of which foods are okay and which ones may be problematic. As you start to experiment with your diet, keep a list of foods that seem to be well-tolerated. (See chapter 2.) The emphasis should be on what you *can* have, not what you *can't*.

Make any changes gradually. The bowel is already in a supersensitive state, so making sweeping changes in diet almost always leads to more symptoms. Proceed slowly, one bite at a time, and one food at a time.

Consuming more fiber may be helpful, especially if constipation is a primary symptom. For example, Mary suffered from IBS characterized by constipation. She would go several days without a bowel movement, and when she finally did have one, she was extremely bloated, uncomfortable, and in a lot of pain. She was told that eating fiber would help. Determined to feel better, she decided that eating a lot of fiber would be the way to go. Mary started her day with a bowl of bran cereal, tried to work in some beans for lunch, and made it a point to include a fruit and vegetable at every meal. Needless to say, she felt more bloated and gassy than she did before, and her bowels still didn't move. She wondered what she was doing wrong.

Well, a little fiber goes a long way. It is very important to add fiber to your diet gradually, only two to five grams at a time, and at one meal, not every meal. In addition, when you add a food with fiber, make it a point to add another glass of water to help to move foods through the intestine. Mary now made the following changes to her diet: she added a small amount of a high-fiber cereal mixed in with her cornflakes for breakfast, a fruit *or* vegetable at every meal (instead of both), and a glass of fluid at every meal. She felt much less bloated and uncomfortable, and soon started having regular bowel movements, too.

It is also very important to make mealtimes relaxed and as stress-free as possible. Sit down, turn off the computer, don't answer the phone, and try to concentrate on enjoying your food. Try to unwind before you eat, so eating can be a more pleasant experience. Establish an eating schedule, planning to eat something at regular intervals, instead of skipping meals. Often, when a meal is missed, you may be overly hungry at the next meal and tempted to eat more, which may make your symptoms worse.

PAIN MANAGEMENT

If you are very uncomfortable after meals, try placing a heating pad or towel-wrapped hot water bottle on your abdomen. The warmth may help to lessen abdominal spasms and decrease pain. If bloating is one of your symptoms, wear comfortable, loose-fitting clothes while you eat to reduce the discomfort.

Some people find that relaxation techniques such as biofeedback, hypnotherapy, and deep breathing techniques can help with pain management. Progressive muscle relaxation can help you learn how to calm your gut. Exercises such as T'ai Chi and yoga can be very soothing to the gut. Some people find that when they are in pain, but don't need to rush to the bathroom, physical exercise can be an effective diversion. When you exercise, blood circulates to other areas of your body away from the bowel. Exercise may help to normalize intestinal contractions. A pleasant walk, a swim, or even a bike ride may make you feel better.

SUPPLEMENTS TO TRY

There are several supplements that may be of benefit. Some individuals have noticed a decrease in pain with peppermint oil capsules and chamomile tea, but these may not work for everyone. Still, it may be worth a try to see if they are beneficial for you. It is important to experiment gradually, trying one item at a time to see if you notice symptom relief. Some people have found relief with enteric-coated peppermint oil capsules. The dosage is 0.2 ml of peppermint oil three times a day, fifteen to thirty minutes before meals. Peppermint oil may decrease the severity of abdominal pain. *Note:* If you suffer from reflux or heartburn, peppermint oil can worsen these symptoms.

Chamomile may also be useful for decreasing abdominal spasms. To make chamomile tea, cover one tablespoon of the dried herb with eight ounces of boiling water, let stand for five to ten minutes, then strain and drink. The tea can be consumed up to four times a day. If you have hay fever and are sensitive to pollens, however, don't use chamomile!

Some people have found that probiotics can be extremely helpful. Probiotics are friendly bacteria that live in the digestive tract. Antibiotics or gastrointestinal illnesses may decrease the number of probiotics in the gut. Probiotic supplements may help to alleviate the symptoms of IBS. The most effective of these bacteria are Lactobacillus acidophilus, L. reuteri, Bifidobacterium bifidum, L. casei, and L. GG. or very simply acidophilus or bifidum. Make sure you select such products appropriately:

- Select supplements that contain 4 to 10 billion CFUs (colony forming units).
- Check the expiration date.
- Make sure to check the label to see if you need to refrigerate the supplement.
- If you tolerate dairy products, consider yogurt with live active cultures.

PRACTICAL EATING STRATEGIES FOR IRRITABLE BOWEL SYNDROM

Use your food diary to develop your list of acceptable and bothersome foods. Instead of a meal plan, here are a few words of wisdom about eating:

- Identify your problem times of the day, and eat accordingly.
- If you have the most discomfort in the morning, try to eat lighter during that time and enjoy your larger meal at the time when you feel most comfortable.
- If you have a long commute to work, it may be better to wait to eat when you reach your final destination.

- If a child has IBS, he or she may feel more comfortable eating breakfast at school than at home.
- Plan your eating around your activities. If you are having a busy shopping day, you may feel better eating little snacks during the day, then a full meal when you get home.

The good news is that with some changes to diet and lifestyle, you can control IBS. So it is worth your time to identify foods and eating behaviors that cause digestive difficulties. If you are always in a rush and don't respond well to stress, seriously consider taking a stress management class, and adding stress-buster activities to your daily routine. These might include physical activity, meditation, or aromatherapy, among others.

Bottom Line

- Keep a food log to determine potential food "stressors."
- Try to make eating as relaxed as possible.
- Find some productive ways to manage symptoms—through exercise, relaxation, or alternative therapies.

CHAPTER 9

Diverticular Diseases

D r. Jones, a recently retired chemist, was an avid gardener who took great pride in growing his wonderful tomatoes. At a recent routine physical, his doctor suggested a colonoscopy to be on the safe side. When the gastroenterologist came in to review the results of the test, Dr. Jones was informed that he had diverticulosis. The nurse handed him a list of foods to avoid, one of them being the seeds of tomatoes. He was very glum when he left the office, and decided that he might as well give up the tomatoes altogether instead of just being able to eat the outer part. When I spoke at a university wellness lecture recently, Dr. Jones came up afterwards to ask if he really needed to seed the tomatoes. I told him that although many health professionals tell their patients to avoid foods with seeds, the dietary recommendations for diverticular disease do not list tomato seeds as a food to avoid, and that he should go ahead and enjoy the entire tomato. The next day, he came to my office with a bag of tomatoes from his garden. We enjoyed them together.

WHAT IS DIVERTICULAR DISEASE?

Diverticular disease is characterized by the presence of small, bulging, abnormal pouches in the intestinal wall. (A single pouch is a diverticul*um*; multiple pouches are diverticul*a*.) Diverticula can develop not only in the large intestine, but in your throat, esophagus, stomach, and small intestine. They are most likely to form in the sigmoid colon, which is the lower left side of the colon.

Diverticular disease is very common in the United States. It occurs with greater frequency in older persons. Only 10 percent of the population aged forty has it, while it occurs in 50 percent of those over sixty. And practically everyone aged eighty, or older has it.

There are two types of diverticular disease: diverticul*osis* and diverticul*itis*.

Diverticulosis is the condition of having pouches in the large intestine. The diverticula tend to form in weakened areas of the intestinal wall. Pressure inside the colon may push on soft areas along the wall of the bowel, causing these areas to develop outward to form the pouches. Most individuals with diverticulosis do not have any symptoms at all. Other individuals may notice tenderness on the lower left side or muscle spasms in the abdomen. Some can suffer from constipation or diarrhea.

Diverticulitis exists when the diverticula become inflamed or infected. This can happen when a piece of stool gets caught in the diverticula. The stool can interrupt blood flow to the pouch, increasing the likelihood that bacteria can accumulate, resulting in infection. Sometimes the diverticula can tear, and just like cuts anywhere else in the body, can become infected. Many people incorrectly think that nuts, seeds, or kernels should be avoided, because they become trapped in the diverticulum and cause infection or inflammation. But as we have just read, diverticulitis is *not* caused by food getting caught in the diverticulum. Some people with diverticulitis notice mild symptoms such as abdominal cramping, or changes in bowel habits. Others have more pronounced symptoms such as fever, nausea, or severe abdominal pain. It is important to see you doctor if you have serious abdominal pain. Don't ignore the symptoms in the hopes that they will go away, especially if you have a fever.

You may wonder why you ended up with diverticular disease while your friend, neighbor, or other family member may be just fine. Three factors that increase the likelihood of developing diverticula are:

- Straining when going to the bathroom
- Age
- A low-fiber diet

As mentioned earlier, the development of diverticular disease increases with age. Structural changes in the intestine may increase the likelihood of pouch formation. As we get older, our body is less efficient at waste removal. The longer stool sits in the colon, the more pressure is exerted on the intestinal wall, which can also result in the formation of diverticula. One of the benefits of eating a diet with more fiber (fruits, vegetables, grains, dried beans, and peas) is that fiber absorbs water as it moves through the digestive tract. The water makes it easier then for you to eliminate stool. If you don't eat enough fiber, your stool will be more compact, and your body may need to strain to eliminate stool. This pressure can cause the pouches to develop.

DIAGNOSIS

Diverticular disease can be diagnosed by one of the following:

- Colonoscopy. After a patient is sedated, the gastroenterologist inserts a narrow tube into the rectum and through the entire colon. The gastroenterologist views the image of the colon on a monitor to check for the presence of diverticula.
- Sigmoidoscopy. This test is similar to the colonoscopy although

it does not require the patient to be sedated. However, for this procedure only the lowest part of the colon, called the sigmoid colon, and in some cases part of the descending colon, are examined.

- X ray of the colon.

If you have pain in your abdomen and/or fever, the doctor may do the following tests for diverticulitis:

- Press on the abdominal area to check for tenderness
- Blood work to see if you have an elevated white blood cell count
- CT scan to indicate the presence of inflamed diverticula

TREATMENT

The treatment for diverticular disease is a combination of the following:

- Specialized diet to increase fecal mass
- Medications
- Surgery
- Stress management
- Exercise

Diverticular disease often requires making modifications to food intake. In some cases, medications may be used. If you require medications for symptoms, they will most frequently be either pain relievers or antibiotics (if infection is present). Surgery is rarely required, but may be necessary if diverticulum rupture.

If you have diverticulosis, you will find it can often be treated by changes in food and fluid intake. Your doctor may suggest a fiber supplement to help make your stools more bulky, so that you don't need to strain when you eliminate. Regular exercise decreases the pressure on your colon, which reduces the risk of diverticula forming. People who exercise regularly find it easier to eliminate without straining.

While you need to develop bowel habits that are less stressful to your body, it is also important to listen to your body's internal cues. When you feel the need to evacuate, don't delay. Give yourself enough time in the bathroom so that you don't have to force a bowel movement. If you have abdominal spasms, relaxation techniques such as deep breathing or visual imagery may be of benefit. If you have cramps, your doctor may prescribe pain medication.

If you have diverticulitis, you may need to go to the hospital, depending on the severity of your symptoms. Your doctor may prescribe antibiotics to help with the infection. You will need to make short-term changes in your diet such as decreasing your intake of fiber until symptoms subside.

In rare cases, surgery may be performed to remove the diseased part of the bowel. The surgeries performed most often are bowel resection with anastomosis and bowel resection with colostomy.

If you have anastomosis, the diseased part of the bowel is removed, and the remaining portions are joined together so that the stool can pass through normally. If bowel disease is extensive, anastomosis may not be an option, and the surgeon may perform a colostomy, in which an opening in the wall of the abdomen, called a stoma, is formed, so that stool can pass through this opening into a bag worn outside of the body.

THE IMPACT OF DIET

Since one of the main causes of diverticular disease is a low-fiber diet, making changes to your eating pattern may help to prevent the disease from worsening. When people are given a recommendation to modify their diet to help with symptoms or disease management, they often respond enthusiastically and try to make dramatic and rapid adjustments, only to end up feeling worse, not better. Here are some of the things people with diverticular disease tend to do incorrectly:

- Add too much fiber too soon
- Neglect to drink enough fluid when adding fiber
- Take too much of a fiber supplement
- Neglect to drink enough fluid with a fiber supplement
- Eliminate all nuts and seeds, however small, from the diet
- Assume that cooking or chopping fruits and vegetables changes the fiber content

NUTRITION SOLUTIONS

As discussed, it is best to increase fiber in your diet if you have diverticular disease. As fiber is the indigestible carbohydrate in plant foods, it helps to create a stool that is bulkier, decreasing pressure on the intestinal wall and lessening the likelihood of the formation of diverticula. Fiber also helps to speed the movement of stool through the colon. Fiber is only found in fruits, vegetables, nuts, grains, dried beans, and peas. The challenge is to increase fiber gradually to prevent the following:

- Constipation
- Bloating
- Diarrhea
- Gas
- Abdominal cramping

A good rule of thumb is to try to increase your fiber intake by *five grams at a time.* If you are not currently eating much fiber, proceed *slowly.* As a starting point, use your food diary to keep track of what you eat over a few days, and figure out how much fiber you are currently consuming. The following table, which lists the fiber content of common foods, will help you estimate your fiber intake. Note that when choosing fruits and vegetables, peels or skins add to the fiber content.

Fiber Content of Foods

Food	Fiber (grams)
A piece of fruit	3
½ cup of canned fruit	2
½ cup of frozen fruit	2
¼ cup of dried fruit	2
1 cup of raw, leafy vegetables	2
½ cup of cooked vegetables	2
½ cup of canned vegetables	2
½ cup of frozen vegetables	2
6-ounce glass of vegetable juice	2
Baked potato, with skin	2.5
Baked potato, no skin	2
½ cup of dry beans, cooked	7
¼ cup of nuts	3

Read the nutrition facts panel on food labels to find out the fiber content of packaged foods. Make sure to consider the serving size as well when you are figuring out the fiber, since the nutrition information corresponds to the serving size eaten. The illustration shows an example of a food label.

As you start to increase your fiber intake, you may want to start buying a different kind of grain product. When you buy breads or cereals, look at the ingredient list. The words "100% whole grain" should be the first item on this list.

You also may need to consider adding other fiber sources to your diet. Fiber supplements such as Metamucil, Konsyl, Citrucel, Fiber-Con, psyllium capsules, or unprocessed wheat bran are good choices, but be aware that fiber supplements will provide just fiber. High-fiber foods provide other nutritional benefits as well.

The following food diary will give you an idea of how to compute a baseline fiber intake. Make copies of the blank fiber diary that follows the sample. Then you can proceed slowly, meal by meal, to add

Nutrition Facts	
Serving Size 1 cup (228g)	
Servings Per Container 2	
Amount Per Serving	
Calories 90	Calories from Fat 30
	% Daily Value*
Total Fat 3g	5%
Saturated Fat 0g	0%
Cholesterol 5mg	2%
Sodium 280mg	12%
Total Carbohydrate 13g	4%
Dietary Fiber 6g	24%
Sugars 3g	
Protein 3g	
Vitamin A 80% • Vitamin C 60%	
Calcium 4% • Iron 4%	

* Percent Daily Values are based on a 2,000 calorie diet. Your daily values may be higher or lower depending on your calorie needs:

		Calories:	2,000	2,500
Total Fat	Less than		65g	80g
Sat Fat	Less Than		20g	25g
Cholesterol	Less Than		300mg	300mg
Sodium	Less Than		2,400mg	2,400mg
Total Carbohydrate			300g	375g
Dietary Fiber			25g	30g

Calories per gram:
Fat 9 • Carbohydrate 4 • Protein 4

Source: FDA and CFSAN

Figure 7.1–Food label highlighting fiber content

more fiber to your diet. Remember to record all foods eaten and beverages consumed, as well as any supplements you use.

Consider making a schedule to help you achieve your new fiber goals, such as adding five grams each week to your daily fiber intake. For example, eat five grams of fiber each day for the first week. The next week, eat ten grams of fiber each day, and so on, until your daily

Sample Fiber Diary

Time	Food	Amount	Fiber (grams)
7 A.M.	Rice Krispies	1 cup	0.5
	Skim milk	4 ounces	0
	Orange juice	6-oz glass	0
8 A.M.	Water	20-oz bottle	0
9 A.M.	Danish pastry, apple	1	1.3
	Coffee	12-oz mug	0
12 noon	Hamburger on a bun	1	0
	French fries	Small	2.4
	Cola	12 ounces	0
	Ketchup	2 packets	0.4
1 P.M.	Licorice	2-oz package	0
2 P.M.	Water	20-oz bottle	0
6 P.M.	Cheese pizza, thin crust	2 slices	4
	Salad	1 cup	1
	Skim milk	8-oz glass	0
8 P.M.	Pretzels	1 handful	1
	Water	8-oz glass	0
Total Daily Fiber			10.6

Your Personal Fiber Diary

Time	Food	Amount	Fiber (grams)

Total Daily Fiber

fiber intake reaches twenty-five grams for women under age fifty or thirty-eight grams for men under age fifty. For those over age fifty, the daily fiber recommendations are twenty-one grams for women and thirty grams for men. These values reflect the revised Dietary Reference Intakes for fiber as recommended by the Institutes of Medicine Food and Nutrition Board. There is no need to increase fiber significantly beyond this amount; in fact, too much fiber can lead to other digestive symptoms such as diarrhea, gas, or bloating. See chapter 15 for a weekly meal plan to increase fiber.

To help in the process of increasing fiber intake, every time you add a new food with fiber to your diet, add another glass of liquid. This can help prevent constipation. Also, try to include a fiber-containing food at every meal or snack, so that you don't have to overload your evening meal with high-fiber foods to meet the day's quota. Be creative about adding fiber, and mix together different foods. For example, make a sandwich with one slice of high-fiber bread and one slice of white bread, or have three-quarters of a cup of your regular cereal with one-quarter cup of a higher-fiber choice.

If you choose to add bran, make sure you choose unprocessed wheat, or Miller's bran, and start with a very small amount, such as one teaspoon per day. Gradually increase to two tablespoons per day over a six-week period.

FOODS TO CHOOSE FOR DIVERTICULOSIS

If you have diverticulosis, try to increase your fiber intake gradually, using the guidelines listed previously. Although nuts and seeds do not have to be eliminated from your diet, be sure to chew foods well. If you love strawberries, rye bread, poppy seed bagels, cucumber and tomatoes—yes, you can enjoy them. The seeds are too small to get caught in the diverticula, so don't worry. Enjoy!

If you have diverticulosis, it is a good idea to watch overall fat intake. A higher-fat diet usually means the diet is lower in fiber. Try to get into the habit of substituting higher-fat snacks with more fruits, vegetables, and grains using the following suggestions:

Instead of:	*Choose:*
Chips and dip	Bean dip and baked tortilla chips
Chocolate bar	Trail mix of cereal and dried fruit
Cheese and crackers	Peanut butter on celery
Pudding	Low-fat fruit yogurt with lower-fat granola added
Fruit juice	A piece of fruit

FOODS TO CHOOSE FOR DIVERTICULITIS

Depending on the severity of your symptoms, you may need to eat very lightly, or your doctor may recommend a liquid diet or low-fiber diet until your symptoms subside. This type of eating plan is temporary, and is done to give your gut a rest, and to allow time for the inflammation to subside.

A low-fiber diet would consist of the following:

Foods to Choose
- Peeled raw fruits
- Fruit juice, strained or clear, such as apple or grape
- Canned fruits except for prunes
- Low-fiber cooked vegetables, such as asparagus, cauliflower, carrots, okra, onions, and turnips
- Low-fiber raw vegetables, such as green pepper, celery, lettuce, peeled cucumber, and tomatoes
- Tomato products, such as sauce, paste, and juice
- Vegetable juice
- Potatoes without skin
- Low-fiber cereals that are rice- or corn-based
- White bread
- White rice
- Pasta

Foods to Limit
- Nuts
- Seeds, (such as pumpkin, sesame, and sunflower)
- Crunchy peanut butter
- Bran
- Multigrain bread, cereal, or crackers
- Whole grain bread, cereal, or crackers
- Whole wheat pasta
- Brown rice
- Dried beans
- Spinach
- Blackberries and raspberries
- Dried fruit
- Coconut

The low-fiber diet is only to be followed for a short period of time. Once you feel better, you should start to gradually increase your fiber intake again.

Bottom Line

Controlling diverticular disease is a matter of being consistent with proper bowel habits and food choices. Diverticulitis is an acute disease, which means that you may need to make temporary changes in eating to allow your body a chance to heal, but once you improve, you should go right back on a maintenance eating plan to keep your gut healthy and decrease your risk of future diverticula forming. Try to do the following on a daily basis:

- Take enough time. Don't rush when you need to move your bowels.
- Don't strain.
- Add in fiber gradually, and be consistent with fiber intake.
- For added benefit, emphasize food sources of fiber over supplements.
- Make sure you drink enough fluids.

Celiac Disease

J anet, a high school math teacher, had been having more frequent episodes of stomach pain, bloating, and diarrhea over the
past year. She was always hungry, but kept losing weight, even
though she was eating more. Finally, she felt so tired and weak that
she decided to see her doctor. On his recommendation, she stopped
using dairy products, but she still felt terrible, and continued to lose
weight. Then she had read an article about some people who have
digestive symptoms when they eat certain grain products. Janet
went back to her doctor, who decided to run additional tests. He
confirmed a diagnosis of celiac disease and told her she would have
to go on a gluten-free diet. Janet called me to find out what that
meant, and to help her put together a meal plan she could live with.

June, CEO of a dot com company, has always been a very high-
energy person. She traveled frequently for her job, both nationally
and internationally. Over the past few months, she has been increas-
ingly fatigued, finding it very difficult to get through the day without taking a nap. She has also been suffering with migraines, which
she never had before. She decided to see her doctor, who ran tests
and discovered that she was anemic. June raised the question of
possible food sensitivities, and asked her physician if it was possible

that she was allergic to certain foods. Although she did not have any gastrointestinal symptoms, diagnostic tests confirmed that June had celiac disease. June was worried that she would not be able to follow the diet because of her travel schedule. Her physician recommended that she contact a registered dietitian for help in developing a meal plan.

WHAT IS CELIAC DISEASE?

Celiac disease, also known as celiac sprue, gluten intolerance, or gluten sensitive enteropathy, is an autoimmune disease that damages the villi, or fingerlike projections of the small intestine. If you have celiac disease, your body is not able to handle gluten, a protein found in wheat, rye, and barley. If you eat a food with gluten, the body reacts in an inappropriate way, causing the cells of the small intestine to respond abnormally. This results in inflammation in the intestinal lining, which can cause the villi in the small intestine to disappear leading to the body's inability to absorb nutrients well. In children and adults, celiac disease can affect growth and can cause deficiencies of iron, calcium, folic acid, and the fat-soluble vitamins A, D, E, and K. In adults, these changes in calcium and vitamin D levels cause a decrease in bone mineral density. Celiac disease can also cause anemia.

Celiac disease has become more common. The rate of occurrence of celiac disease is as follows:

- General population: 1 in 130
- Children with symptoms: 1 in 35
- Adults with symptoms: 1 in 30
- First-degree relatives (grandparents, aunts, uncles): 1 in 12
- Second-degree relatives (cousins): 1 in 13

Celiac disease is the most common genetic disease in Europe, and is increasing in prevalence in the United States. It is rarely found in Africa or in the Far East. Recent studies have confirmed that 5 percent of children with juvenile diabetes in the United States also have celiac disease.

The good news is that celiac disease can be controlled through diet. A gluten-free diet reverses unhealthy changes in the intestine, and can also improve nutrient absorption. Once you stop eating gluten, the intestinal lining starts to heal itself within three to six days. For children with celiac disease, full improvement can take up to one year, but in adults, full recovery can take up to five years.

SYMPTOMS AND DIAGNOSIS

Celiac disease doesn't manifest the same in everyone. Up to 50 percent of those with celiac disease never have gastrointestinal symptoms, or any symptoms at all. Some individuals develop a skin rash, called dermatitis herpetiformis, and others may notice mood changes. If you are symptomatic, you may experience one or more of the following :

Classic Symptoms
- Abdominal pain
- Abdominal bloating
- Cramps
- Diarrhea
- Abnormally-colored or foul-smelling stools
- Constipation
- Excessive gas
- Chronic fatigue
- Muscle wasting
- Weight loss

Nongastrointestinal Symptoms
- Breathlessness
- Anemia
- Migraines

- Infertility
- Bone pain
- Dental changes
- Delayed growth (in children)
- Changes in behavior
- Learning challenges

DIAGNOSIS

Your gastroenterologist may do a biopsy, in which a tiny piece of the small intestine is analyzed to see if the villi have been damaged. In addition, celiac disease is screened for with a blood test, which detects the presence of anti-endomysial, antigliadin, or transglutaminase (tTg) antibodies. Individuals with celiac disease tend to have higher levels of these antibodies in their blood.

TREATMENT

The goal of treatment is to allow the intestines to heal, improve nutritional status, and to prevent further complications. It is very important to treat celiac disease. If left undiagnosed, or if you continue to eat gluten-containing foods, you can cause more damage to the intestinal villi. Left untreated, celiac disease can increase the risk for the following health problems:

- Lymphoma and adenocarcinoma, which are forms of intestinal cancer
- Osteoporosis due to poor calcium absorption
- Miscarriage or fetal abnormalities, due to the mother's inability to absorb nutrients
- Short stature, due to nutrient malabsorption
- Seizures, due to inadequate absorption of folic acid

Untreated celiac disease also increases the likelihood of developing lactose intolerance, so instead of only having to make one set of modifications to your diet, you may now have to make two major ones. (See chapter 11 on lactose intolerance, if you have celiac disease, for dietary information.)

THE IMPACT OF DIET

Diet *is* the treatment for celiac disease, and does result in disease control and symptom relief. Once you eliminate gluten, your body can heal. Although this sounds easy, it can be a difficult diet, especially in the beginning. The following are some of the things that people do wrong:

- Assume that a little bit of gluten-containing foods won't hurt them
- Ignore the diet all together
- Neglect to replace gluten-containing foods with acceptable gluten-free products, resulting in a low-calorie diet that is very boring
- Eat a diet that is too low in fiber, by failing to replace high-fiber grains with additional fruits and vegetables or dried beans and peas
- Selectively eliminate wheat, but include other gluten-containing foods such as rye, barley, spelt, kamut, or semolina

NUTRITION SOLUTIONS

After being diagnosed with celiac disease, you may be overwhelmed with the diet recommendations. A lot of my patients don't like the thought that bread, cereal, pasta, crackers, and cookies will no longer be a part of their eating plan. As a starting point, make copies of the food diary that follows the sample and keep it for a few days to get an idea of your current food choices. Circle the items that you know are gluten-free. If there is a food you are unsure of, refer to the food lists later in this chapter. Mark yes or no in the column labeled gluten-free food.

Sample Food Diary

Time	Food	Amount	Gluten-Free Food Yes/No
7 A.M.	Cream of rice	½ cup dry	Yes
	2% milk	½ cup	Yes
	Orange juice	6-oz glass	Yes
9 A.M.	Apple	1 medium	Yes
11 A.M.	Wheat free crackers	3	No (when looked on label at other ingredients!)
	Water	20-oz bottle	Yes
12:30 P.M.	Cheddar cheese	2 slices	Yes
	Rice cakes	3 large	Yes
	Green grapes	2 handfuls	Yes
	Baby carrots	6	Yes
	Ginger ale	12-oz can	Yes
2 P.M.	Milk Chocolate candy bar	2-oz bar	Unsure
4 P.M.	Caramel corn	A handful	Thought so, but after looking at the bag, found out otherwise
	Water	8-oz glass	Yes
6 P.M.	Chicken with Shake 'N Bake	A breast	Yes for chicken, no for coating
	White rice, boiled with butter and salt	1 cup	Yes
	Broccoli, steamed	1 cup	Yes
	Applesauce, sweetened	½ cup	Yes
	Beer, regular	12-oz can	No
7:30 P.M.	Lemon ice	4-oz container	Yes
8 P.M.	Water	16-ounce glass	Yes

Your Personal Gluten-Free Food Diary

Time	Food	Amount	Gluten-Free Food Yes/No

Next, make a list of all the gluten-free foods you currently eat. Use the information in the Foods to Include section to construct your list. Post this list on your refrigerator, enter it in your PalmPilot or on your computer, and update it frequently with new foods. You will be surprised at how many choices there are.

However, to prevent intestinal damage, you must become an avid food label reader, and be familiar with the different ways gluten can be found in a food. It is not enough to look for the words "wheat-free" on a label; you must look to see that the product is "gluten-free" as well. So it can be a bit complicated. The following foods all contain gluten and must be excluded from your diet:

Wheat	Spelt
Rye	Farro
Triticale	Kamut
Barley	Batter dipped foods
Wheat germ	Foods with hydrolyzed vegetable
Wheat bran	protein and plant protein
Graham flour	Malted milk
Oats	Beer, ale, and lager
Oat bran	Soy sauce made with wheat
Bulgur	Pre-made gravies
Wheat-based semolina	Some salad dressings

Spelt, Farro, and Kamut are other grains that do contain gluten. Triticale is a cross between rye and wheat. Recent studies suggest that oats are gluten-free. However, there is currently an issue of contamination of oat products with wheat, which can create problems for those with celiac sprue.

In addition to the foods just listed, there are some other terms on food labels that may indicate the presence of gluten. To be on the safe side, try to avoid products that contain the following ingredients:

- Hydrolyzed plant protein
- Hydrolyzed vegetable protein
- Starch
- Modified food starch
- Flavorings
- Seasonings
- Dextrin
- Barley malt
- Barley malt syrup

Some seasonings and flavorings can contain gluten, so if they are not clearly identified on the label, be safe, not sorry, and leave them on the shelf.

There are also some nonfood items which can contain gluten. They include:

- Glue of some envelopes
- Postage stamps (buy the self adhesive ones)
- Lipstick
- Some medications

If there is no indication of gluten on the label, to be on the safe side, call the manufacturer to ask if there is gluten in the lipstick you buy, or the medications you take. You can also ask your pharmacist to find out if any of your medications contain gluten. *Do not assume that hypoallergenic is necessarily gluten-free.* Call the manufacturer. It is better to be sure than to be ill.

FOODS TO INCLUDE

Several companies make gluten-free foods. Some offerings include: pizza crust made from rice flour; gluten-free pancake mix; lentil pasta; and gluten-free pretzels.

Also, look for the words "gluten-free" on pastas, crackers, and cookies. These foods are often found in the health food or diet products section of the supermarket. If you can't find a variety of gluten-free products in your local grocery or health food store, you may want to call or e-mail some of the companies listed in the resource section (appendix F) to ask about product availability. You should also talk with your local grocer to see if the store would be willing to order gluten-free products for you.

For a comprehensive list of gluten-free products, you may want to purchase the shopping guide developed by the Tri-County Celiac Sprue Support Group (see appendix F).

The following foods are gluten-free and can be used as desired:

Corn

Rice

Soy flour

Arrowroot

Pea flour

Corn starch

Potato starch

Potato flour

Whole bean flour

Tapioca

Sago

Rice bran

Cornmeal

Buckwheat (although it contains the word "wheat," it is not a grain and is gluten-free)

Flax

Sorghum

Quinoa

Millet

Amaranth

Gluten-free mixes for cookies, pancakes, and breads

Rice and corn pastas

Lentil pasta

Rice-based pizza crusts

Gluten-free cookies

Teff (a gluten-free grain)

Distilled alcoholic beverages

Fresh-cooked fruits and vegetables

Dried beans (not canned)

Fresh-cooked red meats, poultry, fish

Milk

Cream

Buttermilk

Plain yogurt (may contain food starch)

Cheese

Processed cheese

Cottage cheese (may contain food starch)

Ice cream (may contain food starch)

Sherbet

Fruit ice

Egg custard

Whipped toppings

Gelatin desserts

Plain popcorn

Nuts

Tea (but some herbal teas may contain barley)

Coffee

Cocoa

Soft drinks

Plain pickles

Olives

Ketchup

Mustard

Tomato paste

Vinegar (except malt vinegar)

If you enjoy baking, and want to experiment, there are some substitutions you can make for flour. The conversions are as follows:

For 1 cup wheat flour use:

- ½ cup cornstarch
- ½ cup potato starch
- ½ cup arrowroot starch
- ⅔ cup quick cooking tapioca
- 1 cup corn flour
- ¾ cup coarse cornmeal
- 1 cup finely ground cornmeal
- ⅝ cup (10 tablespoons) potato flour
- ¾ cup rice flour

When you use gluten-free grains, you may need to experiment with changing the cooking time, for example, cooking the food longer and at a lower temperature. You also may want to combine flours for better texture in your baked goods. Two excellent recipe resources include: *The Gluten Free Gourmet* series, by Bette Hagman (New York: Henry Holt & Co.) and *Wheat-Free Recipes & Menus: Delicious Dining Without Wheat or Gluten,* by Carol Fenster (Littleton, CO: Savory Palate, 1997.)

EATING STRATEGIES FOR DINING AWAY FROM HOME

One of the challenges if you have celiac disease is what to do when you eat out. Whether eating at school, at work, or in a restaurant, you need to be prepared. I work with a local celiac disease support group, and recently went out to dinner with some of the members. These individuals were very prepared! One by one, they brought out bags of gluten-free rolls and crackers, and asked a lot of questions of the server. She went back to the kitchen to find out what items could be prepared in a gluten-free way. Making special requests like this can save a lot of problems down the road.

When eating away from home, follow these helpful tips:

- Call the restaurant ahead to see if they have gluten-free items, such as rice or potatoes instead of pasta.
- Ask others with celiac disease which restaurants they find to be helpful.
- Order meats that are broiled, grilled, and steamed instead of breaded or floured.
- Don't take anything for granted.
- Ask if the grill is clean and scraped between uses, and if separate pans can be used to prepare your entrée.
- Request salad without croutons.
- Steer clear of soups; gluten is often added as a thickener.
- Order baked or boiled potatoes.
- Be wary of the following preparation methods and ask questions:

    Gravies

    Dredging or dusting (usually with flour)

    Braising

    White sauces

    Bisques

If you have a young child with celiac disease, make sure that you send gluten-free foods with him or her to school or day care. For older children, pack gluten-free snacks in their lunch or knapsacks. Do make sure these foods are clearly labeled for your child. If your child is attending a sleep-over, or is going on a school trip, send a list along with your child with menu items that he or she can have, as well as some clearly labeled gluten-free goodies for munching.

SURVIVAL STRATEGIES

After being diagnosed with celiac disease, you may feel resentful and deprived because many of your favorite foods are now prohibited. If you still want them, even though you know that they can be harmful to your gut, I would strongly recommend that you join a support group. This can be a tremendous resource, and through it you can discover helpful newsletters, recipe swaps, new product updates, and the chance to vent your frustrations. If you can't locate a local group, contact one of the national organizations and get on their mailing list or listserv.

Bottom Line

Celiac disease can be controlled. Eliminating the gluten from your diet helps your gut, so think of the diet as a new adventure in eating, and consider the following:

- Contact a registered dietitian who can help you learn what foods you can and cannot eat, and help you make sure you are getting the nutrients and balance your body needs.
- Experiment with gluten-free products to see what you like.
- Be assertive when you eat out, and consider bringing some "safe" foods with you.
- Take comfort in the fact that you can control this disease by what you choose to eat.

CHAPTER 11

Lactose Intolerance

Jake, an African American football player, was recently diagnosed with a stress fracture in his foot. When asked about his typical diet, he responded that he never eats dairy products because they make him feel very gassy and send him right to the bathroom. Yet one of the recommendations his doctor had made was to boost calcium intake to help his fracture heal. Jerome didn't want to take the calcium supplements because he was afraid they would bind him. He came to my office confused as to what he should do to increase calcium in his diet. He did agree to try adding dairy products, although on a limited basis and in very small amounts. A few weeks later, he came back to see me very surprised. He was now able to drink a glass of milk, or eat a bowl of cereal, without dashing to the bathroom. He had just assumed that he could never use dairy products because other members of his family were not able to use them, and because he had had a reaction to them in larger amounts.

The problem with avoiding dairy products if you don't need to is that you eliminate a valuable source of calcium, protein, and other minerals from your diet. So if you believe you are having lactose-related problems, be sure *not* to self-diagnose, because you may be eliminating valuable foods from your diet for no reason.

WHAT IS LACTOSE INTOLERANCE?

Lactose is the sugar in dairy products that is broken down by the enzyme lactase, which is produced by the body. If there is not enough lactase present, the body cannot digest lactose. If there is not enough lactase, when undigested lactose reaches the colon it is broken down by bacteria and hydrogen gas is released. This is referred to as lactose maldigestion. Luckily, it does not produce digestive problems in most adults. Lactose maldigestion may occur in about 25 percent of the U.S. population and 75 percent of the world's population. Recent research has suggested that there may be more people who are lactose maldigesters who do not exhibit any gastrointestinal symptoms and who are not truly lactose intolerant (those who do have gastrointestinal symptoms). Jerome, and many others like him, are surprised to find out that one can learn to tolerate dairy products.

True lactose intolerance refers to the gastrointestinal symptoms that can occur when there is not enough of the enzyme lactase to digest the lactose in foods. The symptoms can include:

- Gas or bloating
- Diarrhea
- Abdominal pain

Symptoms typically occur within thirty minutes to two hours after eating or drinking lactose-containing foods. Studies have also suggested that the Mexican American, Native American, Asian American, and African American populations have high levels of lactose intolerance. However, more recent studies have demonstrated a high tolerance rate in all of these groups. One in three individuals who think they are lactose intolerant are not.

Lactose intolerance is not the same as a milk allergy. Unless one has what is known as "primary lactase deficiency," where the body does not produce any lactase at all, almost everyone else can learn to tolerate lactose-containing foods. Primary lactase deficiency is very rare.

Lactose intolerance can vary in severity. Some people cannot tolerate any lactose, but more people can actually relearn to tolerate dairy foods. Also, it is important to know that lactose intolerance does not equal dairy intolerance. Dairy foods, such as milk, cheese, yogurt, and ice cream do contain lactose, but often introducing small amounts of these foods over a period of time results in tolerance without symptoms.

PROBLEMS THAT LOOK LIKE LACTOSE INTOLERANCE

If you are allergic to milk, you are allergic to the casein or protein in the milk, not the lactose. Some individuals with milk allergy experience gastrointestinal symptoms, but others may notice skin rashes or nasal congestion. Milk allergy is more common in infants and young children than in adults. If you notice symptoms any time you eat dairy foods, you should contact your doctor.

One other problem can occur with the presence of lactose: lactose nonpersistence is a condition that occurs with aging because of the decline in lactase activity. As we age, our body may not produce as much lactase as when we are younger, especially if we don't include lactose-containing foods regularly in our diet. The old adage, "If you don't use it, you lose it" applies here. If you want to continue to enjoy lactose-containing foods throughout your life, you need to eat them on a regular basis.

If you have had a recent viral infection, you may notice that you are suddenly lactose intolerant. This is usually a temporary situation. As you continue to recover, so will your ability to tolerate lactose-containing products.

DIAGNOSIS AND TREATMENT

The following tests can be used to measure lactose absorption and diagnose lactose intolerance:

- Lactose tolerance test
- Hydrogen breath test
- Stool acidity test

Both the lactose tolerance and hydrogen breath tests start with a lactose challenge: you are given a lactose-containing beverage. When your gut is functioning normally and the body produces enough lactase, lactose will be broken down into glucose and galactose. The liver will convert galactose to glucose, which can enter the bloodstream and raise the blood glucose level. If there is not enough lactase to break down the lactose, blood glucose levels will not rise, and lactose intolerance will be diagnosed.

As mentioned previously, when lactose reaches the gut, bacteria break it down, releasing hydrogen gas. The hydrogen breath test measures the amount of hydrogen gas in the breath. Higher levels of hydrogen in the breath can confirm a diagnosis of lactose maldigestion or lactose intolerance. Certain medications and lactose-containing foods, as well as cigarettes, can also result in increased hydrogen in the breath. The hydrogen breath test uses a beverage that contains fifty grams of lactose (an eight-ounce glass of milk contains twelve and a half grams of lactose). So fifty grams is the equivalent of drinking a quart of milk. Most people would not drink a quart of milk at a time. So even if you have a positive test, you may still be able to tolerate lactose-containing foods, providing you don't eat or drink as much as fifty grams of lactose at one meal. Studies have shown that lactose maldigesters can tolerate up to twenty-four grams of lactose per day (the equivalent of almost three eight-ounce glasses of milk).

The stool acidity test is used to diagnose lactose intolerance in infants and young children. Giving young children a large quantity of lactose at one time, or a lactose load, can cause diarrhea, which can increase the risk of dehydration. The stool acidity test confirms the presence of lactic acid and glucose in the stool, which are produced from undigested lactose.

Treatment of lactose intolerance or maldigestion is based on the severity of symptoms but typically involves one or more of the following:

- Diet changes in the amount and frequency of lactose consumed
- Addition of lactose-reduced foods to the diet
- Supplemental lactase enzymes

THE IMPACT OF DIET

Lactose maldigestion can be controlled through diet. Yet the approach that many individuals take is too drastic, or too exclusionary. The following are some things people tend to do incorrectly:

- Assume that if you think a food or drink will bother you, it will
- Adopt an all-or-nothing approach by either eliminating lactose completely, or eating a lot at one time
- Assume that acidophilus milk is lactose-free (it is not). This milk is often labeled as "Happy milk" or "Smart milk," and people assume it is easier to digest.
- Eat lactose-containing foods on their own
- If severely lactose intolerant, only eliminating dairy foods, forgetting—or not realizing—that lactose can be added to other foods such as lunchmeats, gums, and medications
- Using lactase enzymes incorrectly, such as after a meal instead of before
- Failing to replace needed calcium if dairy foods are eliminated

Most people tend to think of dairy products as the only source of lactose. However, lactose can be added to many nondairy foods. Read labels to check for the presence of lactose in foods. The following table lists food terms that indicate the presence of lactose.

Food Terms That Indicate the Presence of Lactose

Butter	Buttermilk	Cheese	Cream
Chocolate milk	Powdered milk	Evaporated milk	Goat's milk
Ice cream	Ice milk	Low-fat milk	Margarine (except unsalted)
Milk	Milk chocolate	Milk solids	Nonfat milk
Sherbet	Sweetened condensed milk	Whey	Yogurt

The following ingredients do not contain lactose:

- Casein
- Lactalbumin
- Lactate
- Lactic acid

Lactose also can be an ingredient in some nondairy foods, such as powdered coffee creamers or dessert toppings. Lactose is also present in 20 percent of prescription medicines and 6 percent of over-the-counter products. So ask your pharmacist to check the lactose content of your medications

NUTRITION SOLUTIONS

If you are a lactose maldigester, or are lactose intolerant, you will be better able to handle it by *including* it instead of *excluding* it from your diet.

Your ability to digest lactose is influenced by several factors such as:

- Movement of food through the gut
- Lactase activity in the gut
- Presence of bacteria in the colon
- Fermentation of the dairy foods

- Percent of lactose in the food or beverage
- Stomach-emptying time

The good news is that almost everyone can adapt to lactose. If you have been avoiding lactose, you need to proceed slowly in terms of adding it back in to your diet. First, make copies of the food diary that follows the sample and use your food diary to get an idea of what you are currently eating, and to track your symptoms.

Here are some additional suggestions to improve your tolerance of lactose-containing foods:

- Include only one dairy food a day, and gradually increase the amount as the days go by. (A good strategy is to add the equivalent of a maximum of two to five grams of lactose at a time.)
- Only eat one lactose-containing food per meal.
- Start with small amounts of lactose-containing foods (a quarter cup of milk, half an ounce of cheese).
- Start with foods lower in lactose content (see the following table).
- Drink milk, or eat dairy foods, with a meal or a snack, but not alone. This slows the emptying time of the stomach so that lactose does not enter into the intestine quite as quickly, making it less likely that you will experience symptoms.
- Once you are eating several lactose-containing foods a day, space them several hours apart.
- If drinking milk, see if heating the milk improves your tolerance.
- Try lactose-free or lactose-reduced milk if you continue to experience unpleasant symptoms when drinking milk.
- Use lactase enzyme drops if you are drinking milk. However, you must add them at least twenty-four hours before you plan on drinking the milk, or take lactase tablets before you eat dairy foods.
- If you eat cheese, start with cheddar or Swiss, aged cheeses that are naturally lower in lactose than processed cheese, such as Velveeta or cheese spread.

Sample Food Diary

Time	Food	Amount	Activities	Symptoms
8 A.M.	Bagel	1 large	In the car	Felt okay
	Cream cheese	2 Tbsp		
	Coffee, with nondairy creamer	1 container		
	Banana	5-inch		
9:30 A.M.	Cheese danish	1	In a meeting	A little bloated
10 A.M.				Gassy
10:30 A.M.			Bathroom	Diarrhea
11 A.M.	Ginger ale	12-oz can	At desk	Still gassy
12 noon	Bologna sandwich		In office lunchroom	Okay
	Bologna	3 slices		
	Lettuce	2 leaves		
	Wheat bread	2 slices		
	Mayonnaise	1 Tbsp.		
12:30 P.M.			At desk	Gassy
1:30 P.M.			Bathroom	Diarrhea
2 P.M.	Water	4-oz glass	Working at desk	Better
4 P.M.	Milk chocolate candy bar	2-oz bar	Working at desk	Okay
5 P.M.			On the phone in office	Crampy
6 P.M.			Driving home	Gassy
6:30 P.M.			Bathroom at home	Diarrhea
8 P.M.	Oatmeal with brown sugar and a little butter	1 cup	At the kitchen table	Okay
	Tea with lemon	8-oz mug		
10 P.M.			Lying in bed	A little crampy

Note that this person did not eat obvious lactose-containing foods, but the cream cheese, nondairy creamer, cheese Danish, bologna, and milk chocolate all contain lactose, which could have caused the symptoms. Now fill in your own diary.

Sample Food Diary

Time	Food	Amount	Activities	Symptoms

- Try yogurt, which contains bacteria that break down the lactose, and may make such foods easier to digest.
- Buttermilk may also be easier to tolerate, as it is a fermented dairy food, which makes it easier to digest.

You may find that establishing a goal of limiting daily lactose intake to a specific number of grams can be helpful. Every week you can increase your daily lactose intake by five grams. The following example illustrates how you can gradually increase your daily lactose intake. For example, after eating (or drinking) five grams of lactose a day for the first week, try ten grams each day for the second week, up to twenty-five grams daily in the fifth week.

Even after trying this approach, some people may still find they are not able to tolerate any lactose-containing foods at all. Others may be able to tolerate foods that contain small amounts of lactose by including only one item per day, eaten with a meal. Use the following list to help make the choices that are right for you.

Lactose Content of Foods
Lactose-Free Foods

Broth-based soups

Plain meat, fish, poultry (grilled, baked, broiled, steamed)

Peanut butter

Tofu and tofu products

Dried beans

French or Italian bread (or any breads that do not contain milk, dry milk solids, or whey)

Fruit (all)

Vegetables (all but frozen vegetables in a cream, cheese, or butter sauce)

Lactose-free milk

Kosher meats

Potatoes (white or sweet)

Bagels

Pita bread

Pasta

Rice

Noodles

Unsalted margarine

Nondairy creamers (may contain lactose—check label)

Nondairy whipped topping (may contain lactose—check label)

Oil

Fruit ices or sorbet

Gelatin

Jelly, preserves, honey, syrup

Herbs

Spices

Almond milk

Rice milk

Soymilk

Soy yogurt

Soy cheese

Almond milk cheese

Soy-based sour cream

Soy ice cream

Rice milk ice cream

Low-Lactose Foods (0 to 2 grams lactose per serving)

1 to 2 ounces aged cheese, such as Swiss, Cheddar, or Parmesan

1 ounce processed cheese (American)

Butter

Margarine

½ cup regular milk treated with lactase at least twenty-four hours in advance

Lactase-treated milk (Lactaid, Dairy Ease)

2 tablespoons cream cheese

½ cup cottage cheese

½ cup ricotta cheese

High Lactose Foods (5 to 8 grams lactose per serving)

½ cup milk

2 tablespoons powdered milk

¼ cup evaporated milk

3 tablespoons sweetened condensed milk

¾ cup heavy (whipping) cream

½ cup half-and-half

¾ cup sour cream

½ cup white sauce

¾ cup sour cream dip

¾ cup cottage cheese (creamed, regular, or low-fat)

1 cup dry cottage cheese

¾ cup ricotta cheese

3 ounces cheese spread

1 cup ice cream or ice milk

½ cup (4 ounces) yogurt

Some nondairy foods may contain significant amounts of lactose. If you are lactose-intolerant read the labels before buying the following:

Lunchmeats

Hot dogs

Baked goods

Instant potatoes

Instant soups

Beverage mixes

Margarines (except unsalted)

Salad dressings

Candies

Pancake and cake mixes

SUBSTITUTIONS AND MODIFICATIONS

If you had a positive lactose tolerance or hydrogen breath test and have had symptoms after eating only small amounts of lactose-containing foods, you may feel more comfortable taking all lactose-containing items out of your diet. If you do this, you will need to find alternate sources of calcium if you don't use dairy foods. The following is a list of nondairy calcium-containing foods:

Sardines

Canned salmon

Tofu (calcium-fortified)

Shellfish

Turnip greens

Collards

Kale

Dried beans

Broccoli

Calcium-fortified orange juice

Calcium-fortified soymilk

Blackstrap molasses

Almonds

Recipe Modifications

The following substitutes can be used to replace dairy products in recipes:

Instead of	Choose
1 cup whole milk	½ cup soymilk or rice milk and ½ cup water
	or
	½ cup liquid nondairy cream and ½ cup water
1 cup skim milk	½ cup nondairy cream and ¾ cup water
	or
	1 cup lactase-treated milk
½ cup cottage cheese	½ cup soft tofu
1 cup yogurt	1 cup soy yogurt
1 ounce cheese	1 ounce soy cheese
1 tablespoon cream cheese	1 tablespoon mayonnaise

Bottom Line

If you have been eliminating lactose from your diet because you think you are lactose intolerant, you may want to try lactose-containing foods again. After all, even if you are lactose intolerant, you may find that small amounts are not bothersome. Keep these tips in mind:

- Start with a very small amount.
- Proceed gradually, one food at a time.
- Consume dairy products as part of a meal.
- If these foods are still bothersome, try a lactose-reduced product or the enzymes.

Who knows? You may soon find yourself enjoying that milkshake without the worry of needing to find a bathroom, and be proud of the fact that you are including some foods that are good for your bones and body as well. Keep in mind, too, that if dairy is not going to be part of your diet, be creative and try some of the other delicious options to fuel your gut and support your bones.

CHAPTER 12

Gas and Bloating

Anne, a computer instructor in close contact with her students all day, wanted to make sure she had fresh breath. On average, though, she had to consume an entire package of mints daily to keep her breath fresh. She also noticed frequent episodes of gas, bloating, and loose stools. She came to see me because her intestinal discomfort was so irritating and distracting, and because the embarrassment she felt due to the gas prevented her from doing her job successfully.

She was surprised to learn that the very thing she was taking to keep her mouth fresh was the source of her pain and embarrassment. Once she cut out the mints, the symptoms went away. She also found that drinking more water during the day kept her mouth moist and her breath fine.

WHAT CAUSES GAS AND BLOATING?

Intestinal gas is produced in the large intestine from bacteria that break down carbohydrate-containing food, especially bran, dried beans, and cabbage family vegetables. Passing gas is a very normal occurrence for the body. Actually, we tend to pass gas, or flatus, about ten times per day. (Women tend to pass gas seven times a day; men are a little more active, at about twelve times per day.) While gas is a normal and harmless part of the digestive process, it is considered socially unacceptable.

SYMPTOMS

The most frequent symptoms of gas include:

- Belching
- Flatulence
- Abdominal bloating
- Abdominal pain

Many of us belch. When more air is swallowed than is necessary, belching occurs when air is forced out of the stomach by pressure from the diaphragm. Belching is most likely to occur after meals. It is harmless most of the time, and may be more of a learned nervous habit than anything. Learning how to relax when eating, swallowing less air, and making a concerted effort not to belch can help you to overcome this condition.

Bloating is often due to the fact that the intestine cannot effectively move food and fluid through the gut. Bloating can also be a symptom of irritable bowel syndrome, Crohn's disease, fat malabsorption, or H. pylori, the bacteria that can cause ulcers.

Intestinal gas can produce abdominal bloating, which can be severe enough to be quite painful. The odor of gas can be embarrassing, but it is the pain associated with gas and bloating that is most bothersome.

DIAGNOSIS AND TREATMENT

Your physician may ask you to keep a food and symptom diary. In some cases, gas may be caused by lactose intolerance. If bloating is the primary complaint, you may have other tests done to see if there is inflammation in the gut. If belching is the problem, the physician may do an upper GI series, or X rays of the esophagus, stomach, and small intestine to be sure there is no underlying disorder.

The goal of treatment is to decrease the frequency of symptoms as well as the pain associated with gas and bloating. Managing gas, bloating, and belching requires modification of both food choices and eating behaviors.

Sometimes, medications can be helpful to manage the pain and discomfort, but they are solely for symptom relief. If you use over-the-counter remedies, be aware that some products can actually worsen, rather than help, of help your symptoms.

MEDICATIONS AND SUPPLEMENTS

There are many over-the-counter products advertised to help alleviate gas and bloating. Some of these can be effective, but others may actually make you feel worse. Check with your doctor and dietitian before self-medicating, and keep track of symptoms in your food diary, noting whether they are improving, staying the same, or getting worse. The most effective medications include:

- Charcocaps, or activated charcoal
- Pepto-Bismol (bismuth)
- Antacids containing simethicone, such as Mylanta II, Maalox II, Di-Gel, and GasAid

Activated charcoal may absorb some of the gas so you feel less bloated, but does not seem to be effective in reducing flatulence. Since activated charcoal may interfere with the absorption of medications, take it two hours before or after other medications. Bismuth preparations can help with intestinal gas odor. The bismuth binds with the sulfur in intestinal gas to absorb odors. If you take any bismuth preparation, be careful with herbal preparations, as some herbs can interact with the medication. Hawthorn, ginger, garlic, ginseng, and nettle in combination with bismuth can increase or decrease blood glucose (sugar), which can be a problem, especially for people with diabetes. Gingko, garlic, ginger, and ginseng with bismuth can increase the anticoagulant, or blood-thinning, effect.

Simethicone may help to break up the gas bubbles, so that you feel less bloated, but it does not help with intestinal gas odor.

Some people choose antacids to help with symptom relief. Antacids do not decrease intestinal gas, and products that contain bicarbonate or carbonate may actually make gas worse, so avoid taking them at all costs.

THE IMPACT OF DIET

It is important for you to discover which foods and eating habits cause you to feel more gassy and bloated, and to work on eliminating those items from your eating plan. Patients with good intentions in trying to find solutions to get rid of gas may actually make themselves feel worse. Here are some of the strategies to *avoid*:

- *Loading up on gas-decreasing products* (Gas-X, Phazyme, Beano). If you want to try these, experiment with only one product, and follow the dosing directions on the package. Don't be disappointed if the symptoms aren't resolved. These products don't work for everyone.
- *Skipping meals.* Because they are so starved by the time they finally sit down, most people end up overeating. This excess causes more gas and bloating.
- *Eating too much of a certain food.* If you do not regularly eat cabbage, and yet you sit down to a big bowl of cabbage soup one night, your gut may pay the price all night long.
- *Eating a lot of fatty foods.* A high-fat meal of pepperoni pizza, or fried chicken and fried potatoes, may result in a long, painful night.
- *Eating the right foods the wrong way.* People who eat quickly,

gulp beverages, or talk while eating swallow more air, which can lead to more gas and bloating.

NUTRITION SOLUTIONS

Certain foods are more gas-producing than others, but use your food diary to find out what you yourself can tolerate. Some people have problems with broccoli, but do fine with cauliflower. Others find that coleslaw is great, but cooked cabbage is a no-no.

Carbohydrate-containing foods are the culprits here, since bacteria in the colon ferment these foods and cause gas. The small intestine cannot absorb the following types of carbohydrate, which end up in the colon where bacteria metabolize the carbohydrate and produce gas.

- Fiber (in grains, fruits, vegetables, dried beans and peas)
- Raffinose and starchyose (the carbohydrates in dried beans)
- Fructose (the carbohydrate in fruit, honey, and soft drinks)
- Cabbage family foods (broccoli, brussels sprouts, cabbage, cauliflower, kohlrabi)
- Sugar alcohols, such as sorbitol and mannitol, in sugar-free mints and gum, and apple juice

Carbohydrate-containing foods are essential for nutritional well-being, so the solution is not to eliminate these foods altogether. You need to make your own list of items that work for you. Sometimes, eating a little less of a bothersome food can prevent symptoms. Make copies of the food diary that follows the sample and use your food diary to help you determine what you can tolerate. Be sure to record supplements as well as foods eaten, and pay attention to your eating habits, not just what you eat. It is important to note that protein- and fat-containing foods do not produce as much gas, although eating a high-fat diet may make you feel more uncomfortable because these foods stay in the stomach for a longer period of time.

Sample Food and Symptom Diary

Time	Food	Amount	Activities	Symptoms
9 A.M.	Bran muffin Latte	1 large Large	At coffee shop	Felt okay
10 A.M.			In the car	Gassy
11 A.M.	Sugar-free gum	3 sticks	Running around doing errands	Bloated and gassy
12:30 P.M.	Salad with peppers, cucumbers, garbanzo beans, and tuna and a whole grain roll Diet soda	 12-oz can	In a restaurant	Abdominal pain
1 P.M.			At home	Very bloated
3 P.M.	An apple		On the computer	Needed to unbutton pants
6 P.M.	Baked fish with an ear of corn and broccoli	1 piece of fish and ½ cup broccoli	At dinner table	Very uncomfortable
7 P.M.	Water and Pepto-Bismol	8-oz glass		Uncomfortable
8 P.M.				Feeling better

Your Personal Food and Symptom Diary

Time	Food	Amount	Activities	Symptoms

The following foods are more likely to cause symptoms:

- Dried beans
- Broccoli, brussels sprouts, cabbage, cauliflower, kohlrabi
- Bran
- Cucumbers
- Carbonated beverages
- Sugar alcohols such as sorbitol, mannitol, and xylitol, which are in sugar-free gums and mints, jams, and apple juice
- Wheat
- Oats
- Corn
- Lactose (if you are lactose intolerant)
- Fatty foods (fried meats and vegetables, doughnuts, cream sauces, oily sauces)
- Melons

In addition to changing food choices, the following supplements may be helpful:

- Beano
- Chlorophyll
- Nutra Flora

Beano is an enzyme that breaks down the indigestible carbohydrates in foods such as beans, dried fruits, and cabbage-family vegetables before they reach the colon so that less gas is produced. Beano is available in tablets or in drops. While tablets need to be taken *before* you eat, the drops can be added to food right before, or as you are ready to eat (but cannot be added to food that is steaming hot as heat destroys the enzyme, and thus the effectiveness of the supplement). Chlorophyll may be helpful with fecal odor, but be aware that it may turn your stools green. Nutra Flora is a fructo-oligosaccharide, which is a carbohydrate. It may reduce odor, but may also cause gas and bloating.

Supplements That Can Increase Symptoms

There are several products advertised to help with gastrointestinal health (or that are used for symptom relief for diseases or problems that are not related to the gut) that can actually *increase* gas or bloating. If you use any of the following, be aware that they may contribute to your symptoms. Try eliminating the items on this list that you use on a regular basis, and see if your symptoms subside.

Products	*Symptoms*
Bone meal	Gas and bloating
Borage oil	Gas and bloating
Calcium	Gas and bloating
Evening primrose oil	Gas and bloating
Fructo-oligosaccharides	Gas and bloating
Glucomannan	Gas and bloating
Lactulose	Gas
Pectin	Gas
Probiotics	Gas
Psyllium husk	Gas and bloating
S-adenosyl-methionine	Gas
Turmeric	Gas

Eating Behaviors That Can Cause Gas and Bloating

Sometimes, even when you make an effort to decrease gas- or bloat-producing foods in your diet, you may still have symptoms. You also need to look at your eating habits. The following eating habits may contribute to your discomfort, and you may feel better by trying not to do them:

- Chewing gum
- Gulping foods

- Eating while talking
- Using a straw
- Sucking on candies or lollipops
- Drinking soda

If your child suffers from gas or bloating, try to decrease the number and frequency of use of gas-producing foods in the diet, and remind him or her not to engage in the behaviors on the above list.

If your baby suffers from gas, refrain from the following feeding strategies, which can make your infant more uncomfortable.

- Allowing the baby to nurse on an empty bottle (more air is swallowed)
- Allowing the infant to nurse from a bottle with a stiff nipple or one with too small an opening
- Failure to bring the baby to an upright position after feeding

OTHER FACTORS THAT CONTRIBUTE TO GAS AND BLOATING

In addition to eating behaviors, other lifestyle factors that can contribute to symptoms include smoking and ill-fitting dentures.

Smokers may experience more gas and bloating because of the tendency to inhale more air when smoking. If you wear dentures, it is very important to make sure they fit well. Ill-fitting dentures can cause you to have difficulty chewing, and you may take in more air as a result. Have your dentist check to ensure a proper fit, and remember, that the dentures you receive at age sixty will probably not fit you well when you are in your eighties.

In addition to decreasing your intake of gas-producing foods and gas-producing behaviors, try to adopt gas-decreasing strategies. The following recommendations may help you to feel more comfortable:

- Make changes gradually.
- Introduce new foods slowly and one at a time.
- Start with a small amount of a food.
- If you use dried beans, soak them first, drain and rinse, and then cook in fresh water.
- If you use canned beans, drain the liquid they are canned in and rinse well before using.
- Lentils and chickpeas are less gas-producing than white or black beans.
- If you have lactose intolerance and gas is one of your symptoms, try a lactase enzyme product (See chapter 11).

Bottom Line

Intestinal gas, bloating, and belching are usually a result of food choices and eating behaviors. All of the over-the-counter medications are useless if you don't try to work on what you eat and how you eat. For maximum gut comfort, try to do the following regularly:

- Take time to eat.
- Eat slowly and with small bites.
- Eat with your mouth closed.
- Sip, don't gulp.
- Make one eating change at a time.
- Eat smaller amounts of food at one sitting.
- Keep track of your food tolerances and bothersome foods.

CHAPTER 13

Nausea and Vomiting

A ngela, newly pregnant, was having trouble keeping food down. She had two little ones at home, and was always in the kitchen preparing food for them, or so it seemed. By the end of the day, she was usually feeling so nauseated that she would just go to bed without eating. Her obstetrician was very concerned because Angela continued to lose weight, and he suggested that she talk to a registered dietitian to help her find some acceptable food choices to support a healthy pregnancy.

Adam was recently diagnosed with prostate cancer. He was treated with a combination of radiation therapy and chemotherapy, which took care of the tumor but unfortunately did a number on his digestive tract. His wife called to ask if there was anything she could give him that would help with the nausea and vomiting.

WHAT CAUSES NAUSEA AND VOMITING?

Nausea and vomiting are symptoms that can occur in diseases, in response to treatments, or as a result of medication or supplements. The major concern is that prolonged nausea and vomiting can lead to:

- Inadequate food intake
- Dehydration (with vomiting)
- Electrolyte loss (with vomiting)

The electrolytes sodium and potassium are very important for maintaining fluid balance, muscle function, and cardiovascular function. If electrolytes become depleted through reduced food intake caused by nausea, or through vomiting, it is important to replace them immediately.

TREATMENT

The goals of treatment are to help decrease the frequency and severity of nausea and vomiting. It is also important to maintain optimal fluid balance and nutritional status, although this can be a challenge when the thought of eating or drinking is unappealing. So there are times when medications are used, especially if symptoms are severe. But most often, the dietary treatment involves food and fluid choices as well as making changes to your eating environment.

THE IMPACT OF DIET

If you are nauseated, the last thing you probably want to do is eat or drink. The body still needs to be nourished, however, and often the choices you make can result in worsening of symptoms, or diet inadequacy. Here are some mistakes people make when they are nauseated or vomiting:

- Drink a lot of carbonated beverages (Ginger ale does not always settle a stomach, and the carbonation may make you feel worse.)
- Eat sweet foods such as gelatin or fruit ices. (Highly sweetened foods may be more nauseating.)
- Forget to drink fluids, which can result in dehydration.
- Forego eating all together.

- Try to eat hot foods. (The odor may nauseate you more.)
- Try to eat too quickly, to get meals over with in the hopes of stopping the nausea.

NUTRITION SOLUTIONS IF YOU HAVE NAUSEA

When you are nauseated, you may find the following foods to be more tolerable:

- Toast.
- Crackers.
- Yogurt.
- Sherbet. (Lemon, lime, or orange sherbert are less sweet and may be better tolerated.)
- Pretzels.
- Angel food cake.
- Oatmeal.
- Skinned chicken (baked or broiled).
- Canned fruits.
- Clear liquids, sipped slowly. (This includes white grape juice, tea, broth, apple juice, water, sports drinks. If you are also experiencing diarrhea, stay away from apple juice, which can have a laxative effect.)
- Ice chips.

The following food choices may make you feel worse:

- Fatty foods
- Greasy foods
- Fried foods
- Foods with strong odors
- Sweets such as candy, cookies, and cake

In addition to food choices, try to do the following:

- Let your stomach rest after you eat.

- Stay away from strong food odors.
- Let someone else prepare your food.
- Eat foods at room temperature instead of hot.
- Eat lower-fat foods.
- Try a little bit of food at a time, and eat slowly.
- Make sure you drink enough.
- Eat small amounts frequently, for example, every three hours.
- Try fluids between, instead of with meals, which can help to prevent bloating and discomfort.
- Sip liquids through the day. Cold beverages may be easier to tolerate than warm ones.
- If you wake up feeling nauseated, nibble on a cracker or dry cereal before getting out of the bed.
- Relax after meals instead of moving around.
- Sit up for one hour after eating.
- Wear loose-fitting clothes.
- Try relaxation techniques, such as deep breathing, which can be helpful to fight off nausea.

SUPPLEMENTS

Some people find that ginger can settle the stomach. Surprisingly, ginger ale is not the best way to take ginger since the carbonation may make you feel worse. You may want to try grating gingerroot in warm water, to make a tea, or to try chewing on a piece of candied ginger. Discuss with your doctor before experimenting, especially if you are pregnant, or a cancer patient. If you have ulcers, do not take ginger on an empty stomach, as it can worsen symptoms.

Several over-the-counter supplements that are not taken for digestive health can have negative gut consequences. The following supplements may *cause* nausea. If you are taking any of these, and do notice nausea, you may want to discontinue use to see if symptoms subside. Be sure to let your doctor know if you are taking any of these.

Ephedra	EPA
Echinacea	Fish oil
Yohimbe	Iron
Uva Ursi	Medium chain triglycerides
Lactulose	Phosphatidylcholine
5-HTP	Phosphatidylserine
Activated charcoal	Potassium
Bee pollen	Niacin
Borage oil	MSM
Chitosan	Magnesium
Chondroitin sulfate	S-andenosylmethionine
Coenzyme Q10	Shark cartilage
Conjugated linoleic acid	Vitamin B_6
Creatine	Vitamin C
DHA	Zinc

NUTRITION SOLUTIONS IF YOU EXPERIENCE VOMITING

The greatest concern with vomiting is the loss of fluid and electrolytes (the minerals sodium and potassium). It is extremely important to proceed *slowly* in terms of introducing food and fluid after you have vomited. You should not do the following after vomiting:

- Try to eat or drink before the vomiting has subsided
- Try to introduce too much food or liquid, too fast
- Drink carbonated beverages

When the vomiting stops, try these strategies first:

- Start with clear liquids (apple juice, sports drink, warm or cold tea, or lemonade) as follows:

    1 teaspoon every 10 minutes

    Increase to 1 tablespoon every 20 minutes

    Work up to 2 tablespoons every 30 minutes

- Try ice chips, which can keep your mouth moist without giving you too much fluid at a time.
- As you feel able to tolerate foods, try to add in those items that can provide sodium and potassium. Try a small amount, and eat one food at a time. The following foods will provide sodium or potassium, and are also lower in fat content to prevent stomach upset:

For Sodium	*For Potassium*
Broth or bouillon	Nectars
Pretzels	Yogurt
Crackers	Dried fruit
Salt added to food	Citrus fruits or juices
Sports drinks	Banana
Baked potato chips	Baked potato or boiled potato

In addition to food choices, you may find that deep breathing exercises may be helpful in suppressing the urge to vomit.

SUPPLEMENTS

Gingerroot tea or candied ginger may help stop the vomiting, but do not use it if you have ulcers, are pregnant, or are a cancer patient unless you check with your doctor first.

The following list includes supplements that can *cause* vomiting. If you are taking any of these, and have noticed more stomach upset and vomiting, discontinue use to see if you feel better. As always, let you doctor and dietitian know if you take any of these:

Yohimbe
Echinacea
Ephedra
Maté
Ginseng

Black cohosh
Lactulose
5-HTP
Activated charcoal
Borage oil
Bromelain
DMSO
Evening primose oil
Kombucha
Medium chain triglycerides
Potassium
Shark cartilage
Niacin
Vitamin B_6
Zinc

Bottom Line

As uncomfortable as nausea and vomiting can be, for the most part what, when, and how you eat can have a positive effect on symptoms. Try the following to create a positive eating environment:

- Eat foods that are soothing to you.
- Stay away from strong odors. Cold foods often produce fewer odors than hot foods.
- Rinse your mouth out after vomiting.
- Relax before and after meals.
- Eat small amounts of food at a time.
- Choose fluids if the idea of eating is too uncomfortable.

CHAPTER 14

Diarrhea

Mike was a college student who spent spring break on a camping trip. Although he took the necessary precautions in terms of drinking water, when he returned to school, he found that he was going to the bathroom much more frequently, and his stools were runny, not formed. He started feeling dehydrated, and called his parents, who had him see a gastroenterologist. Tests confirmed a parasite was causing the diarrhea. He was put on antibiotics, but was told to stop eating all fruits, vegetables, and grains until the diarrhea subsided. Mike was a vegetarian, and as these were the foods he typically ate, he really didn't want to cut them from his diet. His mother called me and asked if I could provide some further guidance. Mike and I met, and together worked out a meal plan to cut back on fiber-containing foods until the diarrhea subsided, but then to gradually add these foods back again. Mike was willing to modify his diet to allow his gut to rest, knowing that soon he would be able to resume his regular eating pattern.

WHAT IS DIARRHEA?

Normal bowel movements occur from three times per day to three times a week. Diarrhea, which affects children as well as adults, is very common. Diarrhea is a symptom, not a disease, and there are two types: (1) acute, which is short-lived, and often due to an infection; and (2) chronic, which lasts longer than three weeks and may be a symptom of an underlying disorder such as celiac disease, inflammatory bowel disease, or irritable bowel syndrome.

SYMPTOMS

The symptoms of diarrhea are changes in usual bowel movements through an increase in:

- Stool frequency
- Stool fluidity
- Stool volume
  This is often accompanied by:

   Abdominal cramping

   Abdominal pain

   Bloating

   Nausea

   Need to rush to the bathroom

Diarrhea can be caused by any of the following factors:

- Viral infections
- Bacterial infections
- Parasites
- Traveler's diarrhea (chapter 4)
- Reaction to medication, especially antibiotics
- Result of radiation therapy for cancer
- Intestinal disorder

- Caffeine and ethanol, to excess (caffeine relaxes the muscle between the stomach and esophagus, and can stimulate diarrhea)
- Excess fat and sugar intake which can stimulate the digestive tract

DIAGNOSIS

Most cases of diarrhea resolve on their own. However, if you have chronic diarrhea, your physician may want to do some tests to discover the cause. The types of test that you may have include:

- Blood tests
- Stool culture to test for bacteria or other signs of infection
- Foods challenge tests, such as lactose tolerance or food allergy tests
- Sigmoidoscopy
- Colonscopy

For the sigmoidoscopy and colonoscopy, a long narrow tube is inserted into the rectum. This tube is attached to a computer and TV monitor and allows the physician to see the inside of your colon. The sigmoidoscopy focuses on the lower part of the colon, whereas the colonoscopy highlights the entire colon.

TREATMENT

The treatment for diarrhea is designed to:

- Decrease frequency of bowel movements
- Prevent dehydration
- Prevent electrolyte loss (loss of sodium and potassium, which are important for fluid balance and cardiovascular function)

The greatest risk of having diarrhea is becoming dehydrated. This can be life-threatening in infants and young children. If you have diarrhea, or if you have a child with diarrhea, it is important to recognize the signs of dehydration. In adults, the symptoms of dehydration include:

- Thirst
- Decrease in urination
- Fatigue
- Dark-colored urine
- Lightheadedness

In children, the symptoms of dehydration can include:

- Sunken eyes
- Dry mouth and tongue
- Dry diapers for longer then three hours
- High fever
- Listlessness
- Irritability

Treatment can involve the use of medications as well as dietary modifications. The most commonly used medications are:

- Loperamide (Imodium)
- Cholestyramine
- Bismuth (Pepto-Bismol)
- Antibiotics (if the cause of diarrhea is bacterial)

If you are taking any of the medications listed above, be careful about using any herbal supplements, which can interact with these medications. The table on the following page lists potential medication and herb interactions.

THE IMPACT OF DIET

If you or a loved one has ever had diarrhea, you may have been told to try a BRAT diet. This stands for:

<u>B</u>anana

<u>R</u>ice

<u>A</u>pplesauce

<u>T</u>oast

These foods, while not very exciting, can help prevent overstimulation of the bowel, and may slow down the frequency of bowel movements. The problem is that this is a very monotonous, nutritionally unbalanced eating plan. When you have diarrhea, and cut back on, or cut out certain foods, your nutritional well-being is in jeopardy. It can even cause other digestive problems. I encourage you not to do the following:

- Eliminate all fiber.
- Only drink liquids.
- Cut out all liquids (you can become dehydrated).
- Exclude foods with sodium and potassium. These are electrolytes, which can become depleted if you have diarrhea.

Potential Herb and Medication Interactions

Medication	Herbal interaction
Cholestyramine Loperamide	Valerian and kava can increase drowsiness
Bismuth	Hawthorn, ginger, ginseng, nettle can increase or decrease blood glucose
Bismuth Cholestyramine	Gingko, garlic, ginger, ginseng increase the anticoagulant effect

NUTRITION SOLUTIONS

If you are trying to control the frequency of bowel movements, there are certain foods you may need to be cautious with. Sometimes it is the temperature of food, or the amount eaten, that may increase the frequency of bowel movements. If you have chronic diarrhea, you should make copies of the food diary that follows the sample, and keep your food diary to identify problem foods, difficult times of the day, and symptoms. Be sure to record supplement use as well as food intake, and pay special attention to activities you do when you eat, as they may contribute to more frequent trips to the bathroom.

FOODS THAT MAY PRODUCE LOOSE STOOLS

Some foods may produce loose stools. Do not eliminate all of these from your diet immediately, but use your food diary to keep track of those items that seem particularly bothersome, as well as those that seem to be fine.

The following foods may contribute to loose stools:

- Dried beans, corn, vegetables, and cabbage-family vegetables are all high in fiber, which may worsen diarrhea.
- Fruits and juices contain fructose, which can worsen diarrhea.
- Caffeine-containing beverages, such as coffee and tea, can have a laxative effect.
- Hot foods, such as hot beverages and soup, can worsen diarrhea.
- Alcoholic beverages such as beer, wine, and liquor can worsen diarrhea.
- Fatty meats such as bacon, lunch meats, and heavily marbled meats can worsen diarrhea.
- Fried foods, pastries, and chips are high in fat, which can worsen diarrhea.
- MSG, a flavor enhancer, may exacerbate diarrhea.
- Nutrasweet may be a problem for some people.
- Large quantities of nuts or nut butters may worsen symptoms.
- Concentrated sweets can worsen symptoms.
- Dried fruits, such as figs, dates, raisins, and prunes, can have a laxative effect.
- Prune juice can exert a laxative effect.
- Sugar-free gums and mints contain the sugar alcohols sorbitol,

Sample Food Diary

Time	Food	Amount	Activities	Symptoms
8 A.M. to 10 A.M.	Coffee	3 mugs	At home, cleaning	Felt okay
10 A.M.			Vaccuuming	A little bloated
11 A.M.	Coffee	1 mug	On the phone	Cramping
11:30 A.M.			Rushing to the bathroom	Diarrhea
12 noon	Ham and cheese sandwich on a bun	All	Eating on way out the door to pick up kids from daycare	Rumbling in abdomen
12:30 P.M.			Rushing to the bathroom	Diarrhea
2 P.M.	Chocolate chip cookies	2	At table with kids	Okay
	Coke	12-oz can		
3 P.M.			On the phone	Uncomfortable
4 P.M.	Bite of carrot, a handful of pretzels, 2 sips of apple juice		Making dinner	Abdominal pain
5 P.M.				Loose bowels
6 P.M.	Chicken breast	½	Eating quickly to go out grocery shopping	Abdominal pain
	Frozen carrots, steamed	Spoonful		
	Rice	2 spoonfuls		
	Cola	12-oz glass		Okay
6:15 P.M.			Rushing to bathroom	Diarrhea
7 P.M.			Lying on the couch	Pain

Personal Food and Symptom Diary

Time	Food	Amount	Activities	Symptoms

mannitol, and xylitol, which can have a laxative effect.
- Real black licorice (not the candy) can have a laxative effect.

FOODS THAT MAY HELP CONTROL DIARRHEA

- Increase fluids to prevent dehydration, but try to consume fluids between, not with, meals.
- Consume foods and beverages with sodium and potassium:

    Broth (sodium).

    Sports drinks (sodium and potassium).

    Pedialyte (sodium and potassium).

    Bananas (potassium) or banana flakes are a good way to boost potassium, and can be added to hot cereals.

    Nectars (potassium).

    Boiled or mashed potatoes (potassium).
- Eat lower-fiber foods:

    Yogurt (unless you are lactose intolerant).

    Rice.

    Noodles.

    Cream of wheat.

    Grape juice.

    Smooth peanut butter (a small amount at a time).

    White bread.

    Lean meats.

    Cottage cheese.

    Canned fruits in small quantities.

    Vegetables (1 to 2 tablespoons at a time).
- Drink beverages at room temperature, not hot or cold.

SUPPLEMENTS

In addition to food choices that may be bothersome, there are several supplements that are *not* used to help with digestive disorders, but that may have gastrointestinal side effects such as diarrhea. The following supplements may cause more frequent bowel movements, and exacerbate existing diarrhea. Check with your doctor and dietitian before trying any of these.

Supplements That Can Worsen Symptoms

Senna	Chlorophyll
Cayenne	Chondroitin sulfate
Guar gum	EPA
Horse chestnut seed	DHA
Maté	Flaxseed oil
Bee pollen	Glucosamine
Activated charcoal	Lactulose
5-HTP	Guarana
Acetyl L-carnitine	Kola nut
Borage oil	
Bovine colostrum	

Supplements That Can Help
- Psyllium
- Blackberry root bark (used as a tea)
- Probiotics
- Pectin

Although psyllium is often used as a bulking agent for those with constipation, it can be effective in slowing down your bowel movements so that you do not go to the bathroom quite so often. Blackberry root bark contains tannins, which can also help to slow the transit time of stool through the intestinal tract.

Other supplements that may be of benefit include probiotics and pectin. Probiotics may help prevent antibiotic-associated diarrhea.

They are most readily found in yogurt that contains live active cultures such as lactobacillus acidophilus. Look for the term LAC on the label of yogurts in the dairy case; frozen yogurt does not contain LAC! If you are on antibiotics, you need to consume dairy products two to three hours before or after your medications.

Pectin is a form of fiber found in fruits and certain vegetables. Since your tolerance to fruits and vegetables may be lower when you are having a bout of diarrhea, you may want to try to add pectin. Powdered pectin, typically used in making fruit preserves, is sold in grocery stores in the aisle with pudding and gelatin. Certo and Sure-Jel are the most available brands. To help with diarrhea, try drinking one tablespoon of the powder mixed with a quarter cup of lemon water, twenty to thirty minutes before a meal. The powdered pectin is very sweet, and the lemon water helps to cut the sweetness. The type of fiber in pectin may help to slow the emptying of the gut to decrease the urgency.

In addition to food choices, the number of meals is also important. Try to eat smaller, more frequent, meals throughout the day instead of large meals. Also, try to rest after meals. Relaxing after eating can slow peristalsis, the process that passes food through the gut. Make it a point to sit for twenty to thirty minutes after a meal, or try to rearrange meal times so that you don't need to get up and dash out as soon as your plate is empty.

Bottom Line

To prevent complications that can result from frequent bowel movements, try to do the following:

- Identify which foods and fluids are bothersome to you.
- Drink enough fluids apart from meal times.
- Make sure you include foods with sodium and potassium daily.
- Eat less and more often.
- Sit after you eat.

CHAPTER 15

Constipation

J ulie, who had recently turned forty-five, started to notice some changes in bowel habits. She exercised regularly, running four or five times a week, and also ate a diet that included a lot of fruits, vegetables, and whole grains. Yet, now she was having trouble going to the bathroom. She used to move her bowels daily, but lately was eliminating only two or three times a week, and was feeling very uncomfortable. She was also starting to experience more irregular menstrual cycles, and had scheduled an appointment with her gynecologist. Her doctor recommended that she take a laxative in the meantime, but Julie resisted this; because she was a runner, she didn't want to have to worry about needing to find a bathroom when she was out for her run.

The appointment with her gynecologist confirmed that Julie was in perimenopause. As hormonal changes can affect bowel habits, Julie called me to ask if there were any diet changes she could try to take care of the problem. She was still reluctant to take any over-the-counter product to help with constipation, so I had her keep a food record. We reviewed it together, and I recommended that she add a hot beverage in the morning, and to try adding ground flaxseed to her morning cereal. Julie called me two weeks later to say that she felt like herself again.

Normal bowel movements range from a frequency of three times a day to three times a week. True constipation is defined as having dramatic changes in bowel movements, meaning the bowels move less often, or continual, painful straining to eliminate small hard stools. Constipation can lead to hemorrhoids, swollen blood vessels in and around the rectal area, which occur in 50 percent of those over the age of fifty. Triggers for constipation include:

- Inactivity
- Obesity
- Hormonal changes
- Pregnancy
- Irritable bowel syndrome
- Inadequate fluid intake
- Inadequate fiber intake
- Certain diseases and condition including:

    Parkinson's disease

    Multiple sclerosis

    Stroke

    Spinal cord injuries

    Diabetes

    Disorders of the thyroid gland

    Lupus

    Scleroderma

- Certain medications, including:

    Diuretics

    Calcium or aluminum antacids

    Parkinson's medications

    Pain medications with codeine

    Antidepressants

    Antihistamines

Iron supplements

Calcium supplements

- Excessive use of laxatives

SYMPTOMS

If you are constipated, you may notice one or more of the following changes to your bowels:

- Fewer bowel movements than usual
- Straining to eliminate
- Pain when eliminating
- Small, hard stools

DIAGNOSIS

In some cases of constipation, your doctor may want to do tests to determine the cause. The tests may include:

- A physical exam that includes a digital rectal exam
- Blood tests
- Thyroid tests
- A barium enema X ray
- Sigmoidoscopy
- Colonoscopy
- Colorectal transit study
- Anorectal function tests

The barium enema is given after the bowel is clean. This is done by drinking a special solution prior to the test. The barium outlines the colon so that it shows up well on the X rays to determine whether there is an obstruction. For the sigmoidoscopy or colonoscopy, a long, flexible, narrow tube is inserted into the rectum through the anus. For a sigmoidoscopy, the tube is inserted into the lower colon; the tube passes through the entire colon for a colonscopy. The tube is attached to a computer and TV monitor to allow your doctor to view the colon.

The colorectal transit study is used in individuals who have chronic constipation. You will be asked to swallow capsules that contain a substance that is visible on X rays. X rays of the abdominal area are then made over a series of days so that the movement of these capsules can be monitored.

If your anus or rectum is functioning abnormally, you will have an anorectal function test. This can be done through an anorectal manometry test, which measures the anal sphincter muscle tone and contraction. The other test is a defecography, or X ray of the anus and rectum to determine if there are anorectal abnormalities, muscle dysfunction, and whether or not the stool is completely eliminated.

TREATMENT

The goals of treatment for constipation are to improve the frequency of bowel movements and to prevent straining when eliminating. The following strategies may be helpful:

- Eating enough fiber. The Institutes of Medicine Food and Nutrition Board has recently revised the Dietary Reference Intake for fiber. The recommendations are a daily fiber intake of twenty-five grams for women under age fifty and thirty-eight grams for men under age fifty. For those over age fifty, the daily fiber recommendations are twenty-one grams for women and thirty grams for men. See the table on pages 189–191 for the fiber content of foods, and the five-week plan on pages 194–196 for increasing fiber intake.
- Increasing fluid intake.
- Exercising.
- Eliminating when you feel the urge, rather than waiting.
- Taking medications.

Physical activity can stimulate bowel movements, as muscles in the large intestine work better when the rest of the body is exercised. However, you may find that you need a little extra help to stimulate your bowels. There are several different products that can be used. Check with your doctor before you take anything. Medications can also be prescribed to help with constipation.

Over-the-counter medications include laxatives such as Milk of Magnesia or Lactulose, and stool softeners such as Colace or Surfak. Caution is advised, however. Long-term laxative use can damage nerve cells in the colon, and can interfere with the colon's ability to contract, making it harder for you to move your bowels. If you use laxatives regularly, the bowel muscles respond to the signals from the laxative instead of from your body, which can lead to constipation in spite of the fact that most people take laxatives to *help* with constipation. Although some people use mineral oil as a laxative, it is not recommended because chronic use can deplete your body of the fat-soluble vitamins A, D, E, and K.

If you take Colace, be sure not to take it with the herbs hawthorn, ginger, ginseng, or nettle because the interaction between these herbs and the medication can result in fluctuations in blood glucose (blood sugar).

THE IMPACT OF DIET

Even though people with constipation have heard that fiber is important, they do not always add the correct type or amount of fiber. If you increase your fiber intake, it is also necessary to increase fluid as well, or the result can be worsening of the constipation. Here are some things that people do *incorrectly:*

- Add too much fiber too soon.
- Add only one type of fiber, for instance, eating oatmeal every day, instead of including products containing whole wheat or bran. Not all fiber has the same effect on the bowel, and so soluble fiber foods (which dissolve in water instead of absorbing it), such as oats, rye, and dried beans may make you feel more constipated instead of providing relief.

- Add fiber without drinking enough fluid.
- Use a fiber supplement without drinking enough fluid.

NUTRITION SOLUTIONS

Insoluble fiber, the type found in fruit and vegetable skins and wheat bran, is the most helpful for constipation. Fiber adds bulk to the stool, causing it to push against the intestinal wall to force waste through more rapidly. Insoluble fiber also absorbs water to help speed up the passage of waste through the intestines. For adults under age fifty, the daily fiber goal is to consume twenty-five grams for women and thirty-eight grams for men. For those over age fifty, the daily fiber goal is twenty-one grams for women and thirty grams for men. It is important to add the fiber in gradually, adding no more than 5 grams of fiber to the daily total per week. For children ages two to eighteen, the daily recommended number of grams of fiber is their age plus five. For example, a child of age two would require seven grams of fiber a day; a child of ten would require fifteen grams.

The following table lists the fiber content of foods.

Foods with Higher Fiber Content

Food	Serving	Fiber Content (gm)
Cereals and rice		
Bran flakes	½ cup	2.6–3.7
All Bran	⅓ cup	8.8
Puffed Wheat	1½ cups	1.3
Shredded wheat	½ cup or 1 biscuit	2.5
Cheerios	¾ cup	1.2
Wheat flakes	¾ cup	1.8
Oatmeal	½ cup	1.9
Oat bran	½ cup	2.1
Brown rice	⅓ cup	1.6
White rice	⅓ cup	0.5
Dried beans, lentils		
Dried beans	⅓ cup	3.4–3.8
Lentils	⅓ cup	2.6

(continued)

Foods with Higher Fiber Content *(continued)*

Food	Serving	Fiber Content (gm)
Starchy vegetables		
Canned corn	½ cup	6.0
Frozen corn	½ cup	3.4
Corn on cob	6-inch ear	3.6
Lima beans	½ cup	4.4
Peas	½ cup	4.1–5.4
Potato, baked with skin	4 inches long	2.5
Potato, baked without skin	4 inches long	2.0
Acorn squash	¾ cup	4.4
Sweet potato, baked	⅓ cup	0.9
Sweet potato, canned	⅓ cup	1.5
Yam	⅓ cup	1.7
Bread and crackers		
Whole wheat bread	1 slice	1.5
Rye bread	1 slice	1.0
White bread	1 slice	0.5
Pumpernickel	1 slice	3.8
Corn tortilla	6-inch diameter	2.7
Ryekrisp crackers	4	3.0
Whole wheat crackers	4	1.0
Cornbread	2-inch square	1.4
Vegetables		
Asparagus	½ cup	2.1–2.9
Green beans	½ cup	2.0
Beets	½ cup	2.2
Broccoli	½ cup	2.0-2.5
Brussels sprouts	½ cup	3.6
Cabbage, cooked	½ cup	1.6
Cabbage, raw	½ cup	1.5
Carrots	½ cup	1.6–2.4
Cauliflower	½ cup	1.6–2.0
Celery	½ cup	1.3
Greens	½ cup	1.6–3.2
Lettuce	½ cup	0.25
Mushrooms, cooked	⅓ cup	3.1
Mushrooms, raw	½ cup	0.9
Onions	½ cup	2.2

Food	Serving	Fiber Content (gm)
Peppers	½ cup	1.0
Sauerkraut	½ cup	2.4
Spinach, cooked	½ cup	2.1–2.6
Spinach, raw	½ cup	0.7
Tomatoes, cooked	½ cup	1.0
Tomato, raw	1 cup	1.4
Fruits and Juices		
Apple, with skin	1 medium	2.1
Apples, dried	4 rings	3.7
Apple juice	½ cup	0.7
Applesauce	½ cup	2
Apricots	2	1.5
Apricots, dried	7 halves	5.8
Banana	8-inch	1.1
Blueberries	¾ cup	3.7
Dates	2	1.5
Figs	2	6
Fruit cocktail	½ cup	1.4
Grapefruit	½	1.7
Grapes	½ cup	0.7
Kiwi	1	2.3
Mango	½ small	1.5
Melon	1 cup	1.4–1.8
Orange	1 medium	2.0
Orange juice	½ cup	0.4
Peach	1 medium	2.1
Peaches, canned	½ cup	1.5
Pear	1 medium	2.5
Pears, canned	½ cup	2.8
Pineapple, fresh	¾ cup	1.9
Pineapple, canned	⅓ cup	0.7
Plum	1 small	0.6
Prunes	3	4.0
Raisins	¼ cup	2.4
Strawberries	1¼ cups	4.1
Tangerine	1	1.7
Nuts		
Any type of nuts	1 ounce	1–2.2

Sample Daily Food Diary for Fiber Content

Time	Food/ Supplements	Amount	Fiber (gm)
9 A.M.	A banana nut muffin	1 large	1.4
	Diet Coke	12-oz can	0
11 A.M.	Pretzels	1-ounce bag	0.9
	Apple juice	10-oz bottle	0
12:30 P.M.	Tuna salad sandwich on a large roll	3-oz tuna with 2 tbsp mayonnaise	1.3
	Apple	1 medium	3.7
	Iced tea	12-oz bottle	
2:00 P.M.	Peanut butter cups	2	1.6
	Water	6-oz glass	0
6:00 P.M.	Fish sticks	6	0
	Frozen corn, plain	1 cup	4
Total			**12.9 gms**

Your Personal Food Diary for Fiber Content

Time	Food/ Supplements	Amount	Fiber (gm)
Total			

To prevent feelings of fullness or discomfort, try to space fiber-containing foods throughout the day. Make copies of the food diary that follows the sample to keep track of your new fiber intake. If you use any fiber supplements such as Metamucil, FiberCon, or Citrucel, be sure to write those down as well, since they count as part of your daily fiber intake. You can also use the nutrition facts panel of a food label to determine the dietary fiber for foods not on the list.

A good strategy for boosting fiber intake is to start by increasing the fiber content at one meal for the day, and then gradually increase fiber at each meal. The following are some higher fiber choices for meals and snacks:

Breakfast
A higher fiber cereal (check the nutrition facts panel on various brands for the fiber content, and select a cereal with at least 5 grams of fiber per serving)

Oatmeal with fruit added

Whole grain toast with chunky peanut butter

Whole grain waffles with fruit

Lunch
A cup of vegetable or bean soup

A salad with garbanzo beans added and a whole grain roll

A sandwich of hummus on whole grain bread

A black bean burrito

Snacks
Nuts

Dried fruit

Raw vegetables with a bean dip

Popcorn

Whole grain crackers

Dinner
Baked white or sweet potato with skin

Brown rice

Whole wheat pasta

A black bean burger

Baked beans or another dried bean dish

Cooked vegetables, (especially higher fiber choices such as broccoli, cauliflower, cabbage)

Salad

Fruit for dessert

Baked apple or pear

The following is a five-week plan for increasing fiber.

Five-Week Fiber-Increase Menu Plan for a Woman

WEEK 1

		FIBER (GRAMS)
Breakfast	Bagel with creamy peanut butter	0
	Banana	1.1
Lunch	Grilled chicken sandwich with lettuce	Trace
Snack	Apple	2
Dinner	5-ounce piece baked fish	0
	Baked potato, no skin	2
	Green beans, ½ cup	2
	TOTAL FIBER FOR DAY	7.1 grams

WEEK 2

		FIBER (GRAMS)
Breakfast	¾ cup Cheerios with skim milk	1.2
Lunch	Tuna salad on whole wheat bread	3
	Chips	0
Snack	Cereal bar	1
Dinner	Baked chicken breast	0
	⅔ cup brown rice	3.2
	½ cup steamed broccoli	2
	TOTAL FIBER FOR THE DAY	10.4 grams

WEEK 3

		FIBER (GRAMS)
Breakfast	1 cup oatmeal with ¼ cup raisins	6.2
Lunch	Toasted cheese sandwich on white bread	1.0
	Apple	2.1
Snack	Pretzels	0
Dinner	Small steak	0
	½ cup canned corn	6.0
	½ cup cooked carrots	1.6
	TOTAL FIBER FOR THE DAY	16.9 grams

WEEK 4

		FIBER (GRAMS)
Breakfast	½ cup shredded wheat and ⅓ cup BranBuds cereal with skim milk	11.3
	4 ounces orange juice	0.5
Lunch	Grilled chicken on 2 cups lettuce	1.0
	Hard roll	0.5
Snack	Trail mix made of ¼ cup of nuts, ¼ cup of raisins, ½ cup of pretzels	4.4
Dinner	Shrimp stir-fry: 1 cup shrimp, 1 cup mixed Oriental vegetables	4
	over 1 cup white rice	1.5
	TOTAL FIBER FOR THE DAY	23.2 grams

WEEK 5

		FIBER (GRAMS)
Breakfast	2 whole grain waffles with syrup	4
	½ grapefruit	1.7
Lunch	1 cup lentil soup	7
	Turkey sandwich on a bun	0
	Pear	2.5

(continued)

Five-Week Fiber-Increase Menu Plan *(continued)*		FIBER (GRAMS)
Snack	4 Rye Krisp crackers	3
	1 slice Swiss cheese	0
	½ cup baby carrots	1.8
Dinner	2 cups pasta with ½ cup marinara sauce	3
	1 cup spinach salad	1.3
	1¼ cups strawberries with nondairy topping	4.1
	TOTAL FIBER FOR THE DAY	28.4 grams

Here are some other dietary strategies that may prove helpful:

- Drink a hot beverage or eat hot cereal thirty minutes before the time you normally would have a bowel movement.
- Try adding unprocessed bran to foods. Start with 1 teaspoon of bran added to cereal.
- Try adding flaxseed to foods. Start with 1 tablespoon of ground flaxseed, or flaxmeal, added to cereal or applesauce.
- Try a few dried or stewed prunes or prune juice.
- Children and adults with constipation may benefit from two or three fig cookies.
- Black licorice may have a bowel-stimulating effect. (This refers to *real* black licorice, available in health food stores, not Twizzlers!)
- Consider a cup of caffeine-containing coffee or tea to start the day. Caffeine may stimulate bowel movements. However, too much caffeine can be dehydrating to the body, so try to keep your caffeine intake to a minimum.
- Try to add a glass of fluid every time you add another high-fiber food to your diet.

THE IMPORTANCE OF FLUIDS

As you add more fiber to your diet, you must be sure to drink enough fluids. Add an extra eight ounces of fluid for every five grams of fiber you add to your diet to prevent the feeling of bloating and fullness that can be caused by extra fiber. The additional fluid will help keep your stools soft, and make it easier for you to eliminate. Remember that as we get older, it can be challenging to get in the fluid the body needs as thirst is blunted with age. You need to remind yourself to drink enough, and, if you are caring for an older individual, you need to encourage him or her to drink an adequate amount of fluid. You should try for a minimum daily fluid intake of half your weight in pounds. Example: For a woman who weighs 140 pounds, the minimum daily amount of fluid would be 70 ounces. This includes all liquids, such as:

Water

Juice

Sports drinks

Carbonated beverages

Milk

Coffee

Tea (including herbal teas)

Fruits and vegetables

Soups

Popsicles

Gelatin

Although regular coffee and tea are liquid, if you only drink one or two cups of regular coffee or tea a day, don't be concerned. But if your caffeine intake exceeds three to four cups a day, you may want to consider adding in some extra fluid, or switching to decaffeinated products.

Although you may not think such things as gelatin desserts and ice pops are liquid, they do count as part of your daily fluid intake. And all fruits and vegetables are 90 to 95 percent water.

FIBER SUPPLEMENTS

Although food sources are the best way to boost your daily fiber intake, there are some supplements that can be helpful as an additional source of fiber, or because they may help with symptom relief. First try to meet your fiber needs through eating a variety of foods, but if you do choose to take fiber supplements, read the label of the product carefully, follow the dosing instructions, and take them with adequate fluid. If you are on medications, check with your physician before taking any of the supplements listed below as some of these supplements may interfere with your medications. (See the table on the following page for further information).

The following may help to alleviate constipation:

- Bulk-forming laxative fiber supplements such as Metamucil, Konsyl, Citrucel, Fiberall, FiberCon, Psyllium
- Chlorophyll
- Aloe juice
- Cascara (short-term use only)
- Senna (short-term use only)
- Flaxseed

Even though cascara and senna are sold as "natural" laxatives, be careful if using them. Aloe juice used as a laxative can cause diarrhea. Cascara and senna can cause nausea and cramping, and can increase water absorption in the colon and stimulate intestinal contractions, resulting in diarrhea. In addition, chronic abuse of senna and cascara can be habit-forming, and can lead to electrolyte and fluid loss.

Flaxseed is derived from the flax plant. You can buy the seed in the supermarket or in health food stores. Flaxseed needs to be ground to be absorbed, so buy it already ground or grind it yourself in a coffee mill or food processor. Since flaxseed can become rancid fairly quickly, keep it in an airtight container in the freezer or refrigerator. If you buy the whole seeds, only grind as much as you will use at one time.

Some supplements taken for constipation may interfere with medications or vitamin supplements. The following table lists supplement-drug and supplement-supplement interactions.

Supplement	Contraindications
Aloe	Interferes with blood pressure medications, cortico-steroids
Buckthorn Cascara	Interferes with anti-arrhythmics, cardiac glycosides, corticosteroids, digoxin Indomethacin decreases the laxative effect of cascara
Flaxseed	Should not be consumed at the same time as medications, as it may delay their absorption
Glucomannan	Can interfere with the absorption of the fat-soluble vitamins A, D, E, K
Horse chestnut seed Lactulose	Interferes with anticoagulant medications Increases the absorption of calcium and magnesium Antacids can decrease the effectiveness of lactulose
Senna	Interferes with anti-arrhythmics, cardiac glycosides and estrogen Indomethacin decreases the laxative effect of senna

Supplements That Can Worsen Symptoms

Some over-the-counter supplements taken for general health maintenance or symptom relief for nongastrointestinal reasons may have some digestive side effects, including constipation. Check with your doctor and dietitian before taking any of these supplements. The following supplements may increase the likelihood of constipation:

- Agrimony
- Goldenseal
- St. John's wort
- Activated charcoal

- Bone meal
- Calcium
- Iron
- Phytosterols
- Phytostanols
- Probiotics
- Shark cartilage

PHYSICAL ACTIVITY

In addition to consuming adequate fiber and fluid, it is also important to be physically active if you want to reduce the symptoms of constipation. When you exercise, you move all muscles of the body, including those of your gut. Get into the habit of moving more regularly instead of sitting for long periods of time. Basically, any exercise that gets you up and moving will work. Choose what you like, from walking to line dancing, and make exercise a regular part of your daily health regime. This will benefit is not just your gut, but your entire body.

Bottom Line

Keeping your colon healthy and regular involves a combination food choices, adequate fluid intake, and physical activity. Try to implement the following strategies:

- Listen to your body, and go to the bathroom when you feel the urge.
- Make it a habit to include a plant-based food, which is full of fiber, at every meal and snack.
- Drink enough fluids, and drink often.
- Do something physical everyday.

CHAPTER 16

The Supporting Cast:
Disorders of the Liver, Pancreas, and Gallbladder

G ail had gained some weight since menopause, and decided to go on a very low-calorie diet of about 500 to 600 calories per day. She was sitting in her office typing a letter one day when suddenly she had a sharp pain in her abdominal region that caused her to double over. The pain got worse as the day went on, moving up to her chest. Her co-workers thought she was having a heart attack and called the paramedics to take her to the emergency room. After tests were completed, her doctor told her that she had gallstones and would need to be on a low-fat diet. Gail was very confused, because she already was on a low-fat, low-calorie diet. She called me because she didn't know what to do.

GALLBLADDER DISEASE

The gallbladder is involved in the storage and secretion of bile, a substance produced in the liver that helps the body digest and absorb fat. When the gallbladder contracts, bile is secreted into the bile ducts where it is transported to the small intestine to assist with digestion. If you don't have a gallbladder, bile from the liver is transported directly to the small intestine.

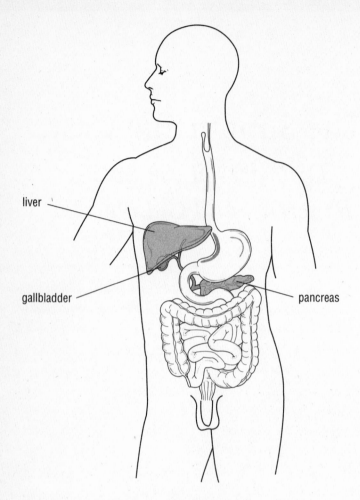

Figure 16.1—More organs in the digestive system

Bile is composed of water, cholesterol, fats, bile salts (which help to digest fats) and bilirubin, a pigment that causes bile and stool to have a brown color. The most common disease of the gallbladder is the development of gallstones, which form when bile hardens. Gallstones are either composed of cholesterol, (cholesterol stones) or bilirubin (pigment stones). About 80 percent of all gallstones are cholesterol stones.

Gallstones form for a number of reasons, including:

- Elevated cholesterol levels
- Being on cholesterol-lowering medications, which increase the amount of cholesterol secreted in the bile, therefore increasing the risk of gallstones
- Infrequent or incomplete gallbladder emptying
- Very-low-calorie diets or fasting, which decreases the contractions of the gallbladder, preventing emptying of bile and increasing the likelihood of stones forming
- Being overweight
- Eating a high-fat, low-fiber diet
- Consuming an inadequate amount of vitamin C
- Physical inactivity
- Having diabetes, since diabetics are more likely to have high triglyceride levels (blood fats), which can predispose one to developing gallstones

Many people with gallstones have no symptoms at all, but between 20 and 40 percent of those with stones will have discomfort or pain. This can be very noticeable after eating fatty foods, such as fried foods or fatty meats, since fat causes the gallbladder to contract. This may cause pain, especially if you have large gallstones.

Gallstones tend to occur more frequently in women than in men, especially in women who have been pregnant, or take birth control pills or hormone replacement therapy. Gallstones also tend to occur more frequently in individuals over the age of sixty. Native Americans and Mexican Americans are more likely to experience gallstones than other ethnic groups.

SYMPTOMS OF GALLSTONES

- Severe, steady pain in the upper abdomen, can sometimes spread to the upper body, resulting in pain that can be mistaken for symptoms of a heart attack. This pain can last from thirty minutes to several hours.

- Indigestion.
- Nausea and/or vomiting.
- Pain in the upper middle back between the shoulder blades.
- Pain under the right shoulder.
- Bloating.
- Belching.
- Gas.

If the following symptoms occur, call your doctor immediately:

- Jaundice, chills, and fever (when the gallstones obstruct a bile duct)
- Jaundiced look to the skin or whites of the eyes
- Stool color change from brown to clay colored

DIAGNOSIS

Gallstones are sometimes discovered through diagnostic tests that are done for another medical problem. They can also be diagnosed through the following procedures:

- Ultrasound
- Cholecystogram
- Endoscopic retrograde cholangiopancreatography (ERCP)
- Blood tests

In the ultrasound test, sound waves will bounce off the gallstones, indicating where they are located. However this test is more precise for detecting the presence of stones in the gallbladder, not those that are located in the bile ducts. For a cholecystogram, the patient is injected with an iodine dye or takes iodine pills the night before the procedure. X rays of the gallbladder can show movement as well as any obstructions within the bile ducts. For ERCP, a long, narrow tube, called an endoscope is swallowed. To make the stones easier to find, dye is injected into the tube, which is connected to a computer and monitor. Blood tests can often determine the presence of infection, jaundice, or pancreatitis, an inflammation of the pancreas.

TREATMENT

Treatment of gallbladder disease is based on the severity of symptoms. If the disease is severe, surgery is performed to remove the gallbladder (cholecystectomy) or to dissolve the gallstones (cholelithiasis). Annually, approximately one-half million cholecystectomies are performed in the United States. If your gallbladder is removed, the liver produces enough bile to digest fat. However, since bile empties directly into the small intestine, instead of being stored in the gallbladder, you may experience more frequent bowel movements in the first few months after surgery, but over time, the gut will adjust.

Cholelithiasis is done by using drugs that dissolve the stones or by using extracorporeal shockwave lithotripsy (ESWL), which breaks the stones into pieces that are small enough to pass through the bile ducts without causing blockages. The medications used to dissolve gallstones include:

- Actigall
- Chenix
- Methy tertiary butyl ether

If surgery is not the course of treatment, the goal is to eliminate the pain by decreasing the secretion of bile from the gallbladder. This is accomplished by eating a low-fat diet, and smaller, more frequent meals. For individuals who are overweight, weight loss can also contribute to symptom relief.

THE IMPACT OF DIET

Although the nutrition strategies for gallbladder symptoms focus on eating a low-fat diet, and eating at regular intervals, many individuals are unclear on what they should be eating. Here are some of the things people do incorrectly:

- Eliminate all fat from their diet
- Only decrease fat *added* to foods, such as butter, mayonnaise, or salad dressing, but still continue to eat higher-fat foods, such as bacon, cheese, and ground meat
- Fail to realize that chips, crackers, and desserts can be a significant source of fat
- Eat large, infrequent meals

NUTRITION SOLUTIONS

The goal is not to eliminate all fat from your diet, but to be careful about how much fat you eat at any one meal. It is a good idea to try to keep your daily fat intake to less than 30 percent of your total daily caloric intake. The following table lists calorie levels and recommended total daily fat intake. But for this table to be truly helpful, it is important to know and estimate your own calorie requirements and make sure you consume an appropriate number of calories per day.

Estimating Daily Calorie Needs

For weight maintenance:

Current weight (pounds) × 13 = number of daily calories for an individual who is sedentary

Current weight (pounds) × 15 = number of daily calories for an individual who exercises two to three times per week

Current weight (pounds) × 17 = number of daily calories for an individual who exercises five times per week

Examples:

A woman who weighs 130 pounds, has a desk job, and does no regular exercise

$$130 \times 13 = 1,690 \text{ calories}$$

A man who weighs 160 pounds and exercise three times a week

$$160 \times 15 = 2,400 \text{ calories}$$

Use the recommended total daily fat intake guidelines in the following table to help you keep track of your daily intake. Then make copies of the food diary that follows the sample to record foods eaten as well as the fat content.

Calorie Level	Total Fat (grams per day)
1,200	40
1,300	43
1,400	47
1,500	50
1,600	53
1,700	57
1,800	60
1,900	63
2,000	67
2,100	70
2,200	73
2,300	77
2,400	80
2,500	83

When it comes to food choices, fats are categorized as those added to foods, and hidden fats. If you are trying to cut down on your fat intake, you should pay attention to both sources of fat. The following strategies may be helpful:

- Read the nutrition facts panel on labels to determine the total fat in foods.
- Trim fat from meats before cooking.
- Remove poultry skin before cooking.
- Use a vegetable spray in place of butter, margarine, shortening, or oil for cooking.
- Skim the fat from the surface of soups.
- Buy low-fat or nonfat dairy products.

Sample Food and Symptom Diary
for Gallbladder Disease

Time	Food	Amount	Fat (grams)	Symptoms
8 A.M.	Cheerios	1 cup	2.0	Felt okay
	2% milk	4 ounces	2.5	
	Banana	½ of 5-inch	0	
9 A.M.	Coffee with half-and-half	10-oz mug 2 tbsp half-and-half	3.4	A little pain
9:30 A.M.	Doughnut, glazed	1	13.7	Nauseous
12 noon	Ham sandwich			Nauseous
	Chipped ham—deli	a small handful	11	
	Hamburger bun	½		
	Mayonnaise	1 tbsp.	11	
	Coke	12-oz can		
1 P.M.	Water	8-oz glass	0	A little queasy
3 P.M.	Snickers bar	1	15	Queasy
6 P.M.	Chicken noodle soup	½ can	2.5	Okay
Total Fat			61	

Your Personal Food and Symptom Diary
for Gallbladder Disease

Time	Food	Amount	Fat (grams)	Symptoms

Total Fat

- Choose lower-fat snack items (but if you are trying to lose weight, don't eat these to excess).
- Increase your intake of fruits and vegetables, which are naturally fat-free and good for you as well.

Food Sources of Fat

Visible Fats (what you add to foods)

Butter

Margarine

Salad dressings

Mayonnaise

Shortening

Oil

Cream cheese

Sour cream

Coffee cream

Cream sauces

Hidden Fats (in the foods we eat)

Dairy products, such as whole or 2% milk, or ice cream

Cheese

Creamed soups

Fatty meats, such as bacon, pepperoni, and sausage

Lunchmeats, such as chipped ham, olive loaf, pimiento loaf, headcheese, bologna, and salami

Ribs

Fish canned in oil

Hot dogs

Prime cuts of meat

Marbled meats (with fat running through the meat)

Fried meats

Fried vegetables such as French fries, onion rings, or fried mushrooms

Tempura-style meats and vegetables

Poultry skin

Nuts and nut butters

Seeds

Chips

Biscuits

Doughnuts

Pastries

Also, be wary of cardamom and peppermint, which can trigger gallbladder contractions resulting in abdominal pain. Try to include no more than one food high in fat at each meal or snack.

Here are some lower fat food choices to include more regularly:

Fruits

Vegetables

Whole grain breads and cereals (except for granola)

Skim or 1% milk

Low-fat yogurt

Cheeses with less than 5 grams of fat per serving

Low-fat cottage cheese

Water-packed canned fish

Turkey breast, from a home-roasted turkey, or deli turkey breast

Skinless poultry

Ground turkey breast

Fish such as cod, flounder, roughy, or sole

Potatoes

Dried beans

Vinegars

Fat-free salad dressings

Vegetable spray

Broth or bouillon

Fruit ice, sorbet, or ice pops

Rice cakes or popcorn

It may also be helpful to increase your intake of vitamin C to meet the recommended dietary requirement of 75 mg per day for women and 90 mg per day for men. vitamin C is needed to break down cholesterol into bile acids, resulting in more cholesterol being excreted, and less being stored to cause stones. Food sources of vitamin C include citrus fruits and juices, strawberries, melons, kiwi, mangoes, and broccoli. In addition, it may be helpful to increase your intake of soluble fiber (oats, fruits, vegetables, barley, dried beans, and peas). Soluble fiber may prevent cholesterol stone formation by increasing cholesterol excretion.

Bottom Line

If you have been diagnosed with gallbladder disease, try to adopt the following strategies:

- Lose weight, gradually, if you are overweight.
- Try to decrease, not eliminate, the amount of fat in your diet.
- Consult a registered dietitian for assistance in helping you develop a low-fat eating plan that you can live with.

PANCREATITIS

The pancreas is a gland behind the stomach (see figure 16.1) that secretes digestive enzymes, which help digest fats, and the hormones insulin and glucagon, which regulate blood glucose. Pancreatitis, a rare disease, is defined as an inflammation of the pancreas. In pancreatitis, the digestive enzymes that normally leave the pancreas through the pancreatic duct to enter the small intestine, stay in the pancreas and irritate the tissues, resulting in inflammation.

There are two forms of pancreatitis: acute and chronic. Acute pancreatitis has a sudden onset, affecting 50,000 to 80,000 individuals yearly. Causes include:

- Alcohol abuse
- Gallstones
- Certain medications
- Trauma to the abdominal region
- Abdominal surgery

Chronic pancreatitis is typically caused by alcohol abuse, although some individuals may inherit the disease. Chronic pancreatitis affects men more than women, and is most common in individuals between the ages of thirty and forty.

SYMPTOMS

The symptoms of acute pancreatitis include:

- Severe abdominal pain that can radiate to the back
- Tender and swollen abdomen
- Nausea
- Vomiting
- Fever
- Worsening of symptoms after eating or drinking alcohol

The symptoms of chronic pancreatitis include:

- Mild to moderate pain
- Nausea and vomiting
- Bloating

- Gas
- Fever
- Worsened pain after eating or drinking alcohol
- Weight loss, due to the fact that fat is malabsorbed
- Diabetes, which can develop if the pancreatic cells that produce insulin are damaged

DIAGNOSIS

If acute pancreatitis is suspected, blood tests are done to detect the following:

- Elevated levels of amylase, a pancreatic enzyme
- Elevated liver enzymes
- Elevated blood glucose
- Elevated blood fats
- Low blood calcium levels

To diagnose chronic pancreatitis, the following tests may be done:

- ERCP (described earlier in the section on gallbladder disease)
- Ultrasound (described earlier in the section on gallbladder disease)
- CAT scan
- Fecal fat test
- Stimulation test

For the CAT scan (or CT scan), X rays of the abdominal region are taken from many angles while the patient is in an X-ray scanner. The fecal fat test involves a challenge test of a very-high-fat diet. This is a way to detect the presence of fat in the stool, to show whether fat is being malabsorbed. In the stimulation test, pancreatic secretions are measured to show whether the pancreas is functioning properly.

TREATMENT

In acute pancreatitis, the goal is to let the pancreas rest, and to restore pancreatic juices. Food is typically withheld for a few days to allow the pancreas time to heal, and nutrients are delivered intravenously. In chronic pancreatitis, pain management and symptom resolution are the primary goals. In addition, digestive enzymes, such as Cotazym, Pancrecarb, Pancrease, or Viokase, may be prescribed to assist in digestion of food. These enzymes replace those that are not being secreted by the pancreas, and are taken with meals. The goals of treatment are to provide symptom relief and to maintain nutritional well-being.

THE IMPACT OF DIET: NUTRITION SOLUTIONS

If you have pancreatitis, the digestive enzymes normally produced and secreted by the pancreas are not available, resulting in decreased absorption of nutrients from foods. Nausea and diarrhea can occur from the malabsorption of nutrients. This is especially true with fats, which can cause diarrhea if not absorbed. As a result, the treatment for pancreatitis is a very-low-fat diet, or approximately forty grams of fat per day.

The following strategies are recommended:

- Eat smaller, more frequent meals.
- Eat a very-low-fat diet. Refer to the following list for foods that are high in fat content, which should be avoided. Also refer to the section on gallbladder disease for lists of foods that contain "hidden" and visible fat.
- Use food labels to monitor fat intake.
- Use fat-free products for cooking, such as vegetable spray, broth, or bouillon instead of oil or spreads.
- Eat enough to maintain body weight by increasing your intake of fat-free cookies, snacks, and beverages, which have lots

of calories but no fat. See the list of fat-free foods, which follows.

Then make copies of the food diary that follows the sample and use it to record foods eaten as well as their fat content.

High-Fat Foods

2% or whole milk

Cheese

Ice cream

Ground meat

Fried meats

Fried vegetables

Bacon, sausage, and pepperoni

Butter

Margarine

Oil

Nuts

Nut butters

Muffins

Doughnuts

Cookies (check the labels for fat content)

Chocolate

Salad dressings

Mayonnaise

Fat-Free Foods

Fruits (all except avocados)

Vegetables

Breads (most are very low in fat)

Cereals (all except granolas, or those with nuts added)

Soda crackers

Bagels

English muffins

Rice

Pasta

Potatoes

Skim milk

Fat-free cheese

Juices

Broth or bouillon

Gelatin

Bottom Line

Pancreatitis can be managed through diet. If you have been diagnosed with pancreatitis, you may need to make changes in your diet to provide symptom relief. Try to do the following:

- Eat a low-fat diet.
- Make sure you eat enough to give your body the calories it needs, by increasing your intake of nonfat items such as grains, fruits, vegetables, beverages, and fat-free snacks.

LIVER DISEASE

The liver (see figure 16.1) is the major filtration system for the body. All nutrients pass through the liver, as well as medications, alcohol, and supplements. The most common liver diseases are hepatitis, which is an inflamed liver, and cirrhosis, which is the development of scar tissue in the liver. Both of these diseases prevent the liver

Sample Food and Symptom Diary for Pancreatitis

Time	Food	Amount	Fat (grams)	Symptoms
9 A.M.	Cinnamon roll	1 large	25	A twinge about 1 hour after eating
	Tea, black	10-oz mug	0	
11 A.M.	Banana	6 inches long	0	Okay
1 P.M.	Pepperoni pizza	2 large slices	Guess about 20 grams each	Pain and nausea
	Cola	12-oz can	0	
3 P.M.	Ginger ale	12-oz can	0	Nauseous
6:30 P.M.	White toast with jelly	2 slices 2 tablespoons	2 0	Okay
	Tea, black	10-oz mug	0	Okay
8:30 P.M.	Orange juice	8-oz glass	0	Okay
Total Fat			67	

Personal Food and Symptom Diary for Pancreatitis

Time	Food	Amount	Fat (grams)	Symptoms

Total Fat

from functioning normally. The liver also can be damaged by any of the following factors:

- Infection
- Parasites
- Obstructions
- Cancer
- Alcohol abuse
- Drug abuse

SYMPTOMS

Although symptoms of liver disease can vary, the effects on nutritional well-being can be profound. Individuals with liver disease often notice the following:

- Decreased appetite
- Nausea
- Vomiting
- Fatigue
- Weight loss
- Food intolerances
- Early feeling of satiety resulting in decreased food intake

TREATMENT

The goals of treatment will differ, depending on the type of liver disease. In some cases, medications will be required. In other cases, a moderate protein diet may be recommended, whereas others may need to restrict sodium and fluid intake. If you have been diagnosed with liver disease, it is critical for you to schedule an appointment with a registered dietitian, who can help you develop a plan to reduce the stress on the liver and promote healing, and also help you maintain nutritional well-being. Contact your local hospital or dietetic group to find a dietitian that you can work with.

THE IMPACT OF DIET: NUTRITION SOLUTIONS

Dietary management of liver disease may involve restricting sodium and fluid intake to prevent edema (fluid accumulation in the extremities) or ascites (fluid accumulation in the abdomen). A moderate protein diet can help prevent the accumulation of nitrogen, a by-product of protein digestion, which can be toxic to the blood and the brain. Restricting sodium and fluid can be difficult, and trying to modify one's own diet may be more detrimental than beneficial. Here are some of the things that people do incorrectly:

- Assume that liquids are the only source of fluid
- Restrict adding salt to food, but continue to eat foods with a high sodium content
- Fail to realize that condiments such as marinades, ketchup, mustard, and relish are all high in sodium content
- Assume that garlic, onion, or celery salt are lower in sodium than garlic, onion, or celery powder
- Forget to count the salt added to boiling water for noodles, or rice
- Fail to drain canned vegetables before heating
- Assume that red meat is high in protein, but chicken and fish are lower in protein
- Forget that grains, vegetables, dried beans, dairy products, and meat are all protein-containing foods
- Cut all protein out of the diet

To determine your fluid or sodium intake, use the following chart as a guide, read food labels, and talk to your dietitian.

The following provides a summary of nutrient guidelines for certain liver diseases.

Nutrient Guidelines for Specific Liver Diseases

Nutrient	Disease		
	Ascites	Edema	Hepatic Encephalopathy
Fluid	1,500 mL	1,500 mL	No restriction
Sodium	2,000 milligrams	2,000 milligrams	No restriction
Protein	No restriction	No restriction	40 grams per day

The following are guidelines for fluid restrictions.

Fluid Restricted Diet

8 ounces of fluid = 1 cup = 240 cc (cubic centimeters)

4 ounces of fluid = ½ cup = 120 cc

1 tablespoon fluid = 3 teaspoons = 15 cc

Fluid Content of Foods

½ cup gelatin, pudding, ice cream, ice milk, sherbet, frozen yogurt	120 cc
12 ounces soda, regular or diet	360 cc
1 cup soup, any kind	240 cc
8 ounces yogurt	240 cc
4 ounces juice, any kind	120 cc
¼ cup syrup	60 cc
8 ounces milk, any kind	240 cc
1 ice cube	30 cc
Popsicle	120 cc

The following provides guidelines for food choices for a sodium restricted meal plan.

Sodium Restricted Diet Guidelines

Lower Sodium Foods (choose more of these)	Higher Sodium Foods (limit these)
Bread	Biscuits
Hot cereals, low-sodium ready-to-eat	Instant hot cereals and most cold cereals

Lower Sodium Foods (choose more of these)	Higher Sodium Foods (limit these)
Cereals (less than 35 grams sodium per serving)	
Unsalted crackers or pretzels	Regular crackers or pretzels
Unsalted chips or popcorn	Regular chips or popcorn
Pasta and rice	Pasta or rice mixes
Potatoes	Instant potatoes or potato mixes
Dried beans or peas	Most canned dried beans
Fresh or frozen meat, poultry, and fish	Canned, smoked, or pickled meats or fish
Unsalted peanut butter	Lunchmeats and regular peanut butter
Eggs	Hot dogs
Unsalted nuts	Nuts
Fresh, frozen, and canned fruits	Dried fruits with sodium added
Fresh, frozen, and low-sodium canned vegetables or tomato products	Regular canned vegetables Regular canned tomato products
Fruit juices and low-sodium vegetable juices	Regular vegetable juices
Milk, yogurt, and low-sodium cheese (less than 35 mg sodium)	Buttermilk, cottage cheese, and cheese
Butter, margarine, mayonnaise, oil, and low-sodium gravies and salad dressings	Bacon, gravies, and regular salad dressings
Low-sodium soup, broth, and bouillon	Regular soup, broth, and bouillon
Gelatin, frozen desserts, and pudding	Pastries, doughnuts, cookies, cake, and brownies
Carbonated beverages, low-sodium diet beverages, seltzer water, coffee, and tea	Diet soda and soda water
Spices; herbs; garlic, onion, and celery powder; vinegar; lemon juice; and pepper	Salt, sauces, and MSG

At times it may be necessary to restrict protein intake to allow the liver to rest. The goal is not to eliminate protein from the diet, but to limit the amount eaten. Protein intake may need to be restricted initially to twenty to thirty grams per day, then gradually increased to sixty grams per day. Here are some tips to help you manage your protein-restricted meal plan.

- Weigh cooked meats to get an idea of the portion size.
- Use a measuring cup for grains, milk, cereals, dried beans, and vegetables.
- Read the nutrition facts panel on labels to determine the grams of protein per serving.
- Be aware that *all* foods—with the exception of fats, fruits, and sweets—contain protein.

The following table lists the protein content of various foods. Note that a three-ounce portion of meat, poultry, or fish is about the size of a deck of cards.

Protein Content of Foods

Food	Amount	Protein (gm)
Beef	3 ounces	21
Pork	3 ounces	21
Veal	3 ounces	21
Lamb	3 ounces	21
Poultry	3 ounces	21
Fish	3 ounces	21
Shellfish	3 ounces	21
Game meats	3 ounces	21
Ground beef or poultry	¾ cup	21
Canned fish	3-oz can	21
Soy burger	1	15–18
Tofu	½ cup	10
Dried beans	½ cup	7–10
Cheese	1 slice	7

Food	Amount	Protein (gm)
Cottage cheese	¼ cup	7
Yogurt	8 ounces	11
Milk	8 ounces	8
Egg	1	7
Egg substitute	¼ cup	7
Peanut butter	1 tablespoon	4
Nuts	¼ cup	10
Ice cream, ice milk	½ cup	4
Pudding, custard	½ cup	4
Bread	1 slice	2
Bagel, English muffin, bun	½	2
Cereal	¾ cup	2
Hot cereal	½ cup	2
Pasta, cooked	½ cup	2
Rice, cooked	½ cup	2
Vegetables	½ cup	1

The following tips will help you manage your meal plan.

- Use a liquid measuring cup to quantify your fluid intake.
- Read the nutrition facts panel on food labels to determine the sodium content per serving.
- Watch condiments and seasonings, which can be high in sodium content.
- Look for the words "salt," "sodium," "baking powder," "baking soda" on labels to indicate the presence of sodium.
- Check foods labeled as "reduced sodium," which may still be high in sodium content.
- Products labeled "instant" are usually higher in sodium.
- When you dine out, order sauces, gravies, and dressings on the side.

Make copies of the food diary that follows the sample, and use it to record your baseline intake of sodium, fluid, and protein.

Sample Food Diary to Determine Baseline Fluid, Sodium, and Protein Intake

Time	Food	Amount	Fluid (cc)	Sodium (mg)	Protein (gm)
8 A.M.	Coffee	12-oz cup	720	8	0
	Orange juice	6-oz glass	180	10	0
	Cornflakes	1 cup	0	304	2.3
	2% milk	4-ounces	120	61	4
10 A.M.	Water	20-oz bottle	600		
12:15 P.M.	Tomato soup	1 cup	240	695	2
	Saltine crackers	6	0	234	1.8
	Grilled cheese sandwich	2 slices American cheese, 2 slices white bread	0	1,082	16.6
2:30 P.M.	Yogurt	6-oz container	180	75	5
	Diet Coke	12-oz can	360	6	0
6:30 P.M.	Baked cod	8-ounce piece, plain, with lemon juice	0	176	52
	Noodles	1 cup, with 2 tsp butter, salted	0	93	7.6
	Canned mixed vegetables	½ cup, drained	0	122	2.1
	Strawberry ice cream	1 cup	240	80	4.2
	Iced tea	12-oz glass	360	15	0
Total			3,000	2,961	97.6

Your Personal Food Diary to Determine Baseline Fluid, Sodium, and Protein Intake

Time	Food	Amount	Fluid (cc)	Sodium (mg)	Protein (gm)

SUPPLEMENTS

Because everything that we eat or drink, including supplements, needs to pass through the liver, you must be especially careful with the use of supplements. Never try any product without first checking with your doctor or dietitian, as many supplements are toxic to the liver.

The following table lists supplements that are toxic, or harmful to the liver and should never be used. These supplements can cause permanent damage to liver cells, or can worsen existing liver disease.

Supplements That Should Not Be Used

Borage leaf	Pennyroyal oil
Chaparral	Uva Ursi
Comfrey	Witch hazel (internally)
Germander	Niacin in megadoses
Groundsel	Vitamin A in large doses
Jin bu Huan	Alcohol

Borage leaf, chaparral, comfrey, germander, groundsel, and Jin bu Huan contain pyrrolizidine alkaloids, which are toxic to the liver. They are available in pills, as tea, and some may be used as a poultice externally. If you use it on broken skin, systemic absorption can cause toxicity to the liver.

Bottom Line

The liver is an essential organ for health and well-being. If you have liver disease, take care of yourself by following these strategies:

• Avoid liver toxins, such as alcohol.
• Be extremely careful with supplement use.
• Contact a registered dietitian to develop a healthy diet that you can live with.

Appendixes

APPENDIX   A

Personal Food, Supplement, and Symptoms Diary

Time	Food/ Supplements	Amount	Activities	Symptoms

Personal Food and Supplements Diary to Record Fiber

Time	Food/ Supplements	Amount	Fiber (gm)

Personal Food Diary to Record Gluten-Free Foods

Time	Food	Amount	Gluten-Free Food Yes/No

Personal Food Diary to Record Dietary Fat Intake and Symptoms

Time	Food	Amount	Fat (grams)	Symptoms

Personal Food Diary to Record Fluid, Sodium, and Protein Intake

Time	Food	Amount	Fluid (cc)	Sodium (mg)	Protein (gm)

APPENDIX   F

Resources

Chapter 4 Resources

American Dietetic Association
1-800-877-1600
www.eatright.org

Home Food Safety website:
www.homefoodsafety.org

Traveler's Hotline—Center for
Disease Control and Prevention
1-888-232-3228
www.cdc.gov.

U.S. Department of Agriculture
14th & Independence Avenue,
S.W.
Washington, DC 20250
Meat and Poultry Hotline:
1-800-535-4555
www.usda.gov

Fight Bac Campaign
Partnership for Food Safety
Education
www.fightbac.org

Chapter 7 Resources

Crohn's and Colitis Foundation
of America, Inc.
1-800-932-2423
www.ccfa.org

Call and ask about a support
group in your area.

Intestinal Disease Foundation
Landmark Bldg., Suite 525
One Station Square
Pittsburgh, PA 15219
1-877-587-9606
www.intestinalfoundation.org

To find a registered dietitian in
your area, contact your local hospital or health department. You can
also contact the American Dietetic
Association for nutrition referrals
and nutrition information.

American Dietetic Association
1-800-877-1600
www.eatright.org

United Ostomy Association
19772 MacArthur Boulevard
Suite 200
Irvine, CA 92612-2405
1-800-826-0826
www.uoa.org

National Digestive Disease
Information Clearinghouse
2 Information Way
Bethesda, MD 20892-3570
301-654-3810
www.niddk.nih.gov

Chapter 8 Resources

Intestinal Disease Foundation
Landmarks Bldg., Suite 525
One Station Square
Pittsburgh, PA 15219
1-877-587-9606
www.intestinalfoundation.org

International Foundation for
Functional Gastrointestinal
Disorders
P.O. Box 17864
Milwaukee, WI 53217
888-964-2001
www.iffgd.org

Chapter 9 Resources

Food and Nutrition Board. *Dietary
Reference Intakes for Energy,
Carbohydrate, Fiber, Fat, Fatty
Acids, Cholesterol, Protein and
Amino Acids.* Washington, D.C.:
National Academy Press, 2002.
http://national-academies.org

Chapter 10 Resources

National Digestive Diseases Information Clearinghouse
2 Information Way

Bethesda, MD 20892-3570
301-654-3810
www.niddk.nih.gov

Celiac Disease Foundation
13251 Ventura Boulevard, Suite 1
Studio City, CA 91604-1838
818-990-2354
www.celiac.org

Gluten Intolerance Group
15110 10th Avenue SW, Suite A
Seattle, WA 98166
204-246-6652
www.gluten.net

The Celiac Sprue
Association/USA, Inc.
P.O. Box 31700
Omaha, NE 63131-0700
402-558-0600
www.csaceliacs.org

American Celiac Society
59 Crystal Avenue
West Orange, NJ 07052-3570
973-325-8837

Canadian Celiac Society
Association
5170 Dixon Road
Suite 203
Mississauga, ON L4W 1E3
Canada
905-507-6208
www.celiac.ca

Tri County Celiac Sprue Support
Group
TCCSSG Shopping Guide
34638 Beechwood
Farmington Hills, MI 48335
248-477-5953

Shelley Case
Gluten-Free Diet: A Comprehen-
sive Resource Guide
Case Nutrition Consulting
1940 Angley Ct.
Regina, SK S4V 2V2,
Canada
www.glutenfreediet.ca

Clan Thompson Gluten Free
Resources
www.clanthompson.com

**Companies That Carry
Gluten-Free Foods**
This is not a comprehensive list,
but will provide a starting point
for obtaining gluten-free products.
Do contact the associations for
more information on where to
obtain gluten-free products.

Ener-G Foods, Inc.
1-800-331-5222
www.ener-g.com

Dietary Specialties
1-888-MENU123
www.menudirect.com

Miss Roben's
1-800-891-0083
missroben@msn.com

Gluten Free Pantry
1-800-291-8386
www.glutenfree.com
Glutino
1-800-363-DIET
www.glutino.com

Gluten-Free Mall
www.glutenfreemall.com

Gluten Solutions, Inc.
737 Manhatten Blvd., Suite B
Manhatten Beach, CA 90266
888-845-8836
www.glutensolutions.com

Chapter 15 Resources
National Digestive Diseases Information Clearinghouse
2 Information Way
Bethesda, MD 20892-3570
301- 654-3810
www.niddk.nih.gov

International Foundation for
Functional Gastrointestinal
Disorders
P.O. Box 17864
Milwaukee, WI 53217
414-964-1799

Intestinal Disease Foundation
Landmarks Bldg., Suite 525
One Station Square
Pittsburgh, PA 15219
1-877-587-9606
www.intestinalfoundation.org

Food and Nutrition Board. *Dietary
Reference Intakes for Energy,
Carbohydrate, Fiber, Fat, Fatty
Acids, Cholesterol, Protein and
Amino Acids.* Washington, D.C.:
National Academy Press, 2002.
http://national-academies.org

Index

acid blockers, 53, 66
acid (pH) probe,
    gastroesophageal reflux
    disease (GERD), 52
Actigall, 205
activated charcoal, 157
acute pancreatitis. *See*
    pancreatitis
alcohol use
    beverage choices, 18
    nutritional well-being, 4
American Dietetic Association,
    2–3
amylase, digestive system, 8
anastomosis, diverticular disease,
    118
anorectal function test,
    constipation, 186
antacids
    gas and bloating, 157
    gastroesophageal reflux
    disease, 53
    ulcers, 66
antibiotics
    diarrhea, 176
    diverticular disease, 117
    inflammatory bowel disease, 78
    ulcers, 66
antidepressants, 104

antispasmodics, 104
anus, large intestine, 12
ascites of liver, nutrition
    solutions, 222. *See also* liver
    disease
azathioprine, 78

barium enema X ray,
    constipation, 186
bathing, stress management, 24
behaviors. *See* eating behaviors
beverages
    constipation, 197–198
    self-management, 17–18
bile
    digestive system, 11
    gallbladder, 202
bile acids, digestive system, 11
bismuth (Pepto-Bismol)
    diarrhea, 176
    gas and bloating, 157
    irritable bowel syndrome,
    104
blood tests
    constipation, 186
    gallbladder disease, 205
    pancreatitis, 214
body weight, gastroesophageal
    reflux disease (GERD), 56

Crohn's disease. *See also*
  inflammatory bowel disease;
  ulcerative colitis
  defined, 74–75
  diagnosis of, 76
  diet, 91–93, 94
  food choices, 20
  relaxation, 25
  supplements, 93–94
  symptoms of, 75–76
cryoprotective agents, 66
cyclosporine, 78

dehydration, diarrhea, 48,
    175–176
diarrhea, 173–183
  case example, 173
  causes of, 174–175
  defined, 174
  diagnosis of, 175
  food-borne illness, 48–49
  food diary, 179–180
  foods causing, 178–181
  foods controlling, 181
  symptoms of, 174
  treatment of, 175–178
  treatment of (diet), 176–177
  treatment of (goals), 175–176
  treatment of (medication),
    176
  treatment of (nutrition),
    177–178
  treatment of (supplements),
    182–183
diary. *See* food diary
diet. *See also* food choices
  celiac disease, 131, 135–137
  constipation, 188–196
  Crohn's disease, 91–93, 94

diarrhea, 176–177, 178–181
diverticular disease, 118–119,
    124–126
gallbladder disease, 205–206
gas and bloating, 158–159
gastroesophageal reflux disease
    (GERD), 55–57
inflammatory bowel disease,
    79–81
irritable bowel syndrome, 102,
    104–106
lactose intolerance, 144–153
liver disease, 221–225
self-management, 14–20
ulcerative colitis, 88–89
ulcers, 68
digestive disorders. *See*
    gastrointestinal disorders
digestive enzymes, small
    intestine, 11
digestive system, 7–12
  esophagus, 10
  generally, 7–8
  illustrated, 9
  large intestine, 12
  mouth, 8
  small intestine, 11–12
  stomach, 10
digital rectal exam, constipation,
    186
diverticular disease, 114–126
  case example, 114
  defined, 115–116
  diagnosis, 116–117
  symptoms of, 115–116
  treatment, 117–126
  treatment (diet), 118–119,
    124–126
  treatment (nutrition), 119–124

irritable bowel syndrome, 99–113
  case example, 99
  defined, 99–100
  diagnosis of, 100–101
  diarrhea, 174
  food diary, 107–108
  studies on, 103
  symptoms of, 100
  symptom triggers of, 101–103
    diet, 102
    hormonal changes, 102–103
    physical activity, 101
    stress, 101
  treatment, 103–113
  treatment (diet), 104–106
  treatment (eating behaviors),
    112–113
  treatment (medication), 104
  treatment (nutrition), 106–110
  treatment (pain management),
    111
  treatment (supplements),
    111–112

jejunum, digestive system, 11

kidney disease, licorice root, 67
kitchen hygiene, food-borne
    illness prevention, 43–44,
    45–46

labeling (of foods)
  dietary fiber, 87, 120, 121
  lactose, 145
  total fat, 92
lactose, food terms indicating
    presence of, 145
lactose intolerance, 140–154
  case example, 140

celiac disease, 131–132
  defined, 141–142
  diagnosis of, 142–143
  food diary, 147–148
  symptoms of, 141
  treatment of, 144–153
  treatment of (diet), 144–153
lactose nonpersistence, 142
lactose tolerance test, 143
Lactulose, 188
large intestine, digestive system,
    12
laxatives, 104, 188
licorice root, cautions about,
    67
lifestyle. *See also* eating behaviors
  gas and bloating, 164
  gastroesophageal reflux disease
    (GERD), 60
  nutritional well-being, 4
  self-management, 22–23
liver
  digestive system, 11
  gallbladder, 201
liver disease
  food diary, 226–227
  overview, 217, 220
  supplements, 228
  symptoms of, 220
  treatment of (diet), 221–225
  treatment of (goals), 220–221
loperamide (Imodium), 104,
    176
lower esophageal sphincter (LES)
  esophagus, 10
  gastroesophageal reflux disease
    (GERD), 51, 56

meal plan, food diary, 33, 36

factors contributing to, 63
food diary, 69–70
symptoms of, 63–64
treatment of, 65–73
treatment of (diet), 68
treatment of (goals), 65
treatment of (medication), 66
treatment of (nutrition), 68, 71–73
treatment of (supplements), 66–68
ulcerative colitis. *See also* Crohn's disease; inflammatory bowel disease
defined, 75
diagnosis of, 76
diet, 88–89
supplements, 89, 91
symptoms of, 75
ultrasound
gallbladder disease, 204
pancreatitis, 214
upper endoscopy
gastroesophageal reflux disease (GERD), 52
ulcers, 64–65

upper gastrointestinal X ray
gastroesophageal reflux disease (GERD), 52
ulcers, 64

variety, food choices, 16–17
vegetables. *See* fruits and vegetables
visualization technique, stress management, 24
vitamins
constipation, 188
digestive system, 11
supplement use, 37
vomiting. *See* nausea and vomiting

water. *See also* beverages
large intestine, 12
small intestine, 11
women
gallstones, 203
irritable bowel syndrome, 102–103

yoga, 23, 111

About the Author

Leslie Bonci, M.P.H., R.D., is a nationally recognized nutrition expert in the area of digestive disorders as well as sports nutrition. She is a national media spokesperson for the American Dietetic Association. Leslie is on the board of the Intestinal Disease Foundation, and works quite closely with the Crohn's and Colitis Foundation of America to provide nutrition expertise in print as well as presentations to patients, family members, and health professionals.

American Dietetic Association

With nearly 70,000 members, the Chicago-based American Dietetic Association is the nation's largest organization of food and nutrition professionals. ADA serves the public by promoting nutrition, health, and well-being.